PRANIC HEALING

PRANIC HEALING

Choa Kok Sui

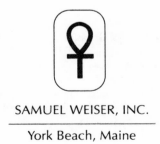

SAMUEL WEISER, INC.

York Beach, Maine

First published in 1990 by
Samuel Weiser, Inc.
Box 612
York Beach, Maine 03910

99 98 97
10 9

Library of Congress Cataloging-in-Publication Data
Choa Kok Sui.
    Pranic healing/by Choa Kok Sui.
        p. cm.
        1. Healing.   2. Vital force.   3. Yoga, Hatha.   I.Title.
RZ401.S84   1990
615.5–dc20   90-38634
                                                    CIP
ISBN 0-87728-713-9
BJ

Typeset in 10 point Galliard by NK Graphics

Printed in the United States of America

The paper used in this publication meets the minimum requirements of the American National Standard for Permanence of Paper for printed Library Materials Z39.48-1984.

"a landmark in the history of psychic healing in our country. No one has attempted a book of this kind and consequence before. . . no one has a grasp of this subject—in theory, experience and application—as thoroughly as he."

—Celso Al. Carunungan, Ph.D.
Chairman of the Board of Regents
University of the City of Manila

". . . offers us a practical and comprehensive guide to cure a variety of ailments: fever and colds, ulcers and stomach disorders, migraine and tension headaches, toothache, lung and breathing problems, arthritis, glaucoma, back pains, heart troubles, disorders of internal organs, muscle pain, high blood pressure, insomnia, and many others. It is not only an effective, simple, and inexpensive form of healing therapy but is also the safest and the most practical. What makes it even more appealing are the instantaneous results one sometimes experiences even after only going through a single session."

—Rolando A. Carbonell, Ph.D.
World Fellow, International Institute of Integral
Human Sciences Montreal, Canada

"I have treated so many patients with Pranic Healing and most of them have responded very well.

"Pranic Healing is indeed simple and easy to learn. At least one member in each family should know Pranic Healing. It is very useful in relieving simple ailments and as well as a form of pranic first aid."

—Manuel M. Fernando, Jr., M.D.

Contents

Level Three: Absent Healing

Level Four: Advanced Pranic Healing

Meditation on the Twin Hearts

The Future of Pranic Healing

Appendices

List of Plates

Acknowledgments

To my Respected Teacher Mei Ling and others for instruction and blessings.

To Mike Nator and others for helping me with esoteric experiments and clairvoyantly monitoring them.

To my wife for assisting me so that I could write this book.

To Dr. Rolando Carbonell, Marilou Guillen, and Lynn Payno for their valuable advice and for editing the work.

To Benny Gantioqui for the air brush paintings and illustrations.

And to all those who gave help and support.

*Dedicated
to my parents,
to my Respected Teachers,
especially
Mei Ling,
and to my two countries,
the Philippines and China.*

A Preview

HAUNTED ARE those who feel they have the gods at their beck and call and daemons on their backs. Clairvoyants say this is not just a feeling but a fact. We all are haunted by two "phantoms"—an inner and an outer aura that follow the contours of the physical body and compose the luminous energy field in which we live and move and have our being. When we sicken, it's because of an energy "leak" in either the inner or the outer aura.

Choa Kok Sui, who has been working with paranormal healing for twenty years, does not believe that any special, inborn healing power is needed to perform paranormal cures. "I am not a clairvoyant nor was I born with any healing ability. If I could learn how to heal effectively, then you can also! All that one needs is the willingness to heal." In fact, his policy is to have every patient learn how to cure him or herself. His purpose is to make "what's considered paranormal healing today quite common and normal a few decades from now." And the cases he cites fascinate us because they sound so commonplace.

A musician named Romualdo, 49, was diagnosed as suffering from cardiac injury and cholesterol deposits in the heart. While undergoing medical treatment, he was urged by his son to try pranic healing at the same time, which he did, under Choa Kok Sui. After several sessions, Choa Kok Sui told him: "You are already cured!" When the musician was inspected by his cardiologist, the latter was astonished to find that the patient had recovered so instantaneously, and without hospitalization. An X-ray disclosed no heart damage; he was fit to work. Romualdo is convinced it was the pranic treatment that hastened his cure.

A housewife, 24, was two months pregnant with her first child when she suffered bleeding and stomach pains. Her doctor thought she might miscarry; the medicine he gave her stopped the bleeding but not the stomach pains. Finally she went to Choa Kok Sui, who treated her only once and for only five minutes. But the pain disappeared immediately, and her pregnancy was not aborted.

A lawyer, 68, had shaking hands, weak knees and chest pains. Ten years of medical treatment failed to stop the spasms and the pains. "Then Choa Kok Sui treated me, praying over me several times. I felt my body becoming lighter, and my muscle being activated. Also, something was being cleansed from my body by some mysterious force. Now I can eat without assistance because my hands no longer shake; I can now walk faster; and I experience chest pains only when I am very tired or emotionally upset."

Do these cases prove that pranic healing works? Choa Kok Sui says that prana, or ki, is the vital energy or life force called *pneuma* by the Greeks, *mana* by the Polynesians, and *ruah* (breath of life) by the Jews. "The healer projects prana into the patient, thereby healing him." There are three major sources of prana. From the sun comes the solar prana that invigorates and that can be absorbed by sunbathing and drinking sun-exposed water, but too much solar prana can harm because it is so potent. From the air comes the ozone prana most effective when acquired through deep slow rhythmic breathing and through the energy centers (called chakras) of the inner and outer aura, which is our ethereal body or envelope. From the earth comes the ground prana that enters through the soles of our feet.

Moreover, says Choa Kok Sui, trees and plants absorb prana from sun, air and ground and exude a lot of excess prana: "Tired or sick people benefit much by lying down under trees. Better results can be obtained by verbally requesting the being of the tree to help the sick person get well. Prana can be projected to another person for healing: people who are depleted tend to absorb prana from those with an excess of it. This is why you may have encountered people who tend to make you feel tired or drained for no apparent reason." Said Jesus: "Someone has touched me, power has gone from me."

The pranic healer must sensitize fingertips and eyes so he or she can "feel" and "scan" the aura (or ethereal body) of the patient and thus verify where the sickness or energy "leak" is. But this requires no clairvoyance or psychic power, according to Choa Kok Sui.

"You do not even have to tense your muscles or exert extraordinary effort when you *will* or *intend*. You don't have to visualize or close your eyes. When you perform with understanding, expectation and concentration, you are already *willing*! The degree of concentration required is not extraordinary. The degree of concentration used in reading a book is sufficient to perform pranic healing." Among the religious, regular meditation is advisable and the treatment should begin with a prayer and invocation.

"Pray for a few minutes any religious prayer you are used to. Then mentally recite the healing invocation: *Lord, make me thy healing instrument. Let my entire being be filled with compassion for others who are suffering. Lord, let your healing and regenerating power flow through this body. With thanks and in full faith!* The invocation should be repeated twice with humility, sincerity, reverence, and intense concentration. Then place your hand on the affected area and mentally recite: *In His name, you are clean, whole and perfect! You are healed! So be it!* Continue the invocation until you feel that the patient will be all right."

Once, suffering from a severe headache, Choa Kok Sui, instead of seeking treatment, experimented by listening to soothing music, and found the headache reduced.

"So, relaxing the mind helps the body heal itself. I have observed that focusing on the pain and trying to remove it makes healing difficult. But ignoring the pain and diverting attention to something pleasant speeds up the rate of healing."

From this he has moved on to the practice of training patients to heal themselves.

"The patients should be instructed to drink energized water and to recuperate under a big tree. Some patients even go to the extent of embracing the tree. Those who are religious should pray regularly, requesting the Lord to make them whole and perfect again. Others who are not the praying type can be taught how to contact spiritual guides through visualizing. For example, they can visualize they're in a beautiful garden among beings of light. The visualization does not have to be clear, just enough to divert their attention from their ailments and discomforts. Their condition will improve; their pain will be alleviated."

Choa Kok Sui has organized this information into a book that's lucid and readable. Even people who tend to shy away from things mystical and unearthly may gain a number of pointers from his practical manual on paranormal healing.

As he says in amen after every session: "With thanks! So be it!"

Nick Joaquin
Philippine Daily Inquirer

Foreword

THERE IS a depth and breadth in pranic healing that is not yet understood by the casual observer. It is a distinct system of healing based on its own philosophy of life and the supreme realization that there is a basic vital energy in the human body which is responsible for the maintenance of health.

Presented here for the first time is a comprehensive study and practical manual by a competent Oriental healer which will throw a new light on the healing process itself. It is, in fact, a pioneering work of historical magnitude, and is based on the author's almost two decades of research and study in esoteric sciences. While this healing approach may astound some orthodox views, its final merit is proven through the efficacy of results in healing. Fortunately enough, with ongoing research efforts and amazing discoveries in the realm of psychic phenomena and paranormal healing, modern instruments are now able to measure and photograph this energy field which exists around the physical organism.

Long before the advent of modern science, ancient sages and healers affirmed the presence of the human aura. In the Bible, reference is made in Genesis to the "breath of life" which holds the very key to human existence, a seemingly mysterious force that animates and sustains life. It has also been affirmed that the movement and quality of circulation, rhythm, and purity of *prana* is what determines the quality of our health, even our emotional states and modes of thinking. We can no longer ignore that nonphysical components and processes within the physical or material dimension exist.

In fact, the more we know about the body, the more we are mystified at its wonderful working precision. No machine, for instance, can repair its own broken parts, but the body does this through the vital energy or *prana* it breathes, the water it drinks, and the food it consumes.

At the present stage of evolution, we are little aware of the pranic forces, and consequently heavily identify ourselves with matter, deluding ourselves into thinking that we are the body. Well-known authority on *Yoga and Medicine*, Dr. Steven Brena, wrote in his book that:

> Man also forgets that matter is nothing else but condensed energy in continuous transformation. He wastes vital energy to feed his senses with a variety of stimulations, born out of an unending chain of material desires. The more he dwells on matter, the more he needs 'fleshly' nutrition to keep himself alive, and the more he burns out oxygen, the less he feels the pranic forces within himself. This situation makes him sink into matter, and with less prana, he becomes depleted.[1]

We certainly owe much to Choa Kok Sui for his many years of research in the study of pranic healing. He is showing us the way to live according to the laws of nature. This is evident in his discussions on karma and the principle of love. It is also in the spirit of reverence and humility that the author infuses a breath of spiritual significance to his work, especially in his chapter on meditation on the two hearts (Illumination Technique).

Written in a simple, direct and straightforward manner and without any elaborate or abstruse language characteristic of scientific and technical or scholarly studies, Choa Kok Sui goes directly to the very core of the principle he is espousing—and proceeds to explain the process of pranic healing, which he asserts most people can immediately learn and experience. You will shortly discover the amazing yet easy-to-follow techniques on healing.

Pranic Healing offers us a practical and comprehensive guide to cure a variety of ailments: fever and colds, ulcers and stomach disorders, migraine and tension headaches, toothache, lung and breathing problems,

---

[1]Dr. Steven Brena, *Yoga and Medicine*. This book is now out of print, but you may be able to find a copy in a used book shop.

arthritis, glaucoma, back pains, heart troubles, disorders of internal organs, muscle pain, high blood pressure, insomnia, and many others. It is not only an effective, simple, and inexpensive form of healing therapy, but is also the safest and most practical. What makes it even more appealing are the instantaneous results people sometimes experience even after only going through a single session.

If he speaks with authority, it is because he has devoted two decades of his life in the study and practice of esoteric sciences, yoga systems, and paranormal subjects. Choa Kok Sui is, however, far from being a reclusive mystic or an ivory tower scientist. He is a rare combination of the practical and the spiritual.

I personally know him as an authentic healer of the first caliber, as a guru (a reluctant one), and above all, as a humanitarian. It is perhaps this deep loving kindness that impelled him to publish this book, which may become one of the most important health care revolutions of this century.

Quantum changes are occurring in all fields of human endeavor. One of the most phenomenal of these changes is happening in the field of healing and spiritual enlightenment. As an observer of the new age phenomenon, I believe that the time has come for sharing the efficacy of pranic healing.

David Spangler, another spokesman of the new age, summarizes the current situation in a quotation from his lecture entitled "Revelation: The Birth of a New Age":

A new world is taking birth. This world already exists and in a sense, its energies are precipitating out into form.

People throughout the world are beginning to attune to this energy, because in their higher consciousness they are already part of that world. They are citizens of it, though they may not know it consciously. Through the power of their lives, in their individual and collective demonstration, they provide precipitation points.

I have strong reasons to believe that this book is one of those significant precipitation points. It will provide a landmark in the field of health and healing which is destined to effect changes in our lifestyle and way of thinking.

I have personally benefited from the tremendous effects of pranic healing. And I fully endorse this technique that I consider a boon and a gift to humanity. As one who has engaged in personal research on the healing arts and human science since 1963, not only in the Philippines but all over the world—I must say that pranic healing is the most unique, though less dramatic, of them all. The drama lies in its effectiveness.

May this book be both a grace and a blessing to you, as it has been to me. And may you experience, too, not only the joy of being healed—but importantly, the *gift of healing* itself—which is extending the frontiers of loving service to everyone.

Rolando A. Carbonell, Ph.D.
World Fellow, International Institute of
Integral Human Science
Montreal, Canada

Preface

THERE ARE many points of view concerning diseases. According to Christian belief, disease has been the scourge of humanity ever since Adam and Eve were driven out of Paradise after they had disobeyed God. Originally, we were disease-free by nature. Disease, therefore, is seen as a punishment for sin. This is one theory or point of view.

Western allopathic medicine on the other hand, holds to the view that disease is caused by such malevolent microscopic creatures as bacteria, germs or viruses which alter our natural physiological functioning or defense mechanisms. Disease can also be caused, according to this view, by emotional stress or psychological problems.

Because disease is believed to be caused either by an infection, an allergen, or a breakdown in physiological functioning, all one has to do is to remove or neutralize the invading mechanism or stress-inducing situation or agent and presto! The patient will be cured. Unfortunately, not all diseases respond to these methods of treatment, despite the impressive advances of modern medical science. As a matter of fact, some medications prescribed by doctors have serious side-effects.

There appears to be a third alternative view, one that has been neglected by modern medical science. I refer here to the energy body that we all have and its crucial role in the causation and treatment of diseases.

The existence of the energy body (sometimes called the etheric double, or vital body) and its intimate interaction with the physical body, are what gives meaning to and effectiveness of pranic healing as described in this book.

"The recognition of the existence of the vital body," as the book *Unrecognized Factors in Medicine*, published by Theosophical Research Centre in London, pointed out, "provides an explanation for the success of such general treatments (as pranic healing), since they tend to restore a ready flow of prana, and the flow of prana, or vital energy, is the chief determining factor for the bio-electric conditions within a living form."

Modern Kirlian photography has shown that disease appears first in the energy or vital body before it manifests itself in the physical body. There is an intimate connection between the two. Therefore, by treating the vital body, we can often effect a cure in the physical body. And this is what *Pranic Healing* by Choa Kok Sui is all about; it is indeed a significant contribution to alternative healing practices.

What makes the book more valuable is the fact that it has a minimum of theory and a maximum of practical and specific advice on how to perform the type of healing advocated by the author. It does not contain any mumbo-jumbo, nor any elaborate ritual which may offend certain religious groups. It is as straightforward as any scientific process should be. It does not intend to supplant orthodox medical treatment, but merely to complement it. This is a handbook which can be used profitably by anyone interested in developing natural healing abilities. I am convinced that this book will be accepted by a wide segment of our society.

Jaime Licauco
President, Philippine Paranormal
Research Society, Inc.

PRANIC HEALING

The most beautiful experience we can have is the mysterious. It is the fundamental emotion which stands at the cradle of true art and science. Whoever does not know it and can no longer marvel, is as good as dead, and his eyes are dimmed.

—Albert Einstein

Introduction

THIS BOOK is a discussion of paranormal healing, not so much on its speculative aspect, but rather more on how and why. The approach in this book is simplified and mechanistic. It is at the same time spiritual. Mechanistic in the sense that all that one has to do is to follow the instructions step by step, and the predetermined results will follow. Spiritual in the sense that, by praying or by invoking, one becomes a divine healing channel. This book teaches, within a week or two, how to heal simple ailments; and within a month or two how to heal difficult cases. One does not have to spend ten to twenty years just to learn how to perform paranormal healing. Nor does one need any special inborn healing power, nor be a clairvoyant to heal. All that one needs is the willingness to heal and to follow the instructions given in this book.

At a very young age I became interested in yoga, psychic phenomena, mysticism, Chinese ki kung (the art of generating internal power) and other esoteric sciences. Because of this interest, I have spent more than eighteen years researching and studying esoteric sciences. I have also been in close association with yogis, healers, clairvoyants, practitioners of Chinese ki kung, and a few extraordinary persons who are in telepathic contact with their spiritual gurus. We have spent several years experimenting to determine the effectiveness and the mechanisms of the healing techniques commonly known and used by healers and students of esoteric sciences. Many of the techniques have been revealed in books by other writers, while some have been rediscovered. Advanced techniques that were privately taught to me are revealed in this book to help uplift the suffering of humanity due to diseases. Many of the advanced healing techniques and concepts were taught to me by my Respected Teacher Mei Ling. I am not a clairvoyant nor was I born with any healing ability. If I can learn how to heal effectively, then you can also!

The instructions have been arranged in such a way that an ordinary person can easily and gradually learn how to perform paranormal healing. Instructions on how to paranormally diagnose a patient without using clairvoyance is also given. For easier and faster understanding, you may want to first scan through the entire book and read the illustrations thoroughly.

The term paranormal healing may not be the proper description. What is considered paranormal healing today may become quite common and normal a few decades from now. This is exactly the purpose of this book: to make paranormal healing quite common in the near future. The appropriate term should be *pranic* or *ki* healing since vital energy or ki is used to heal, and to give proper recognition to its ancient origin and to all esoteric students who have greatly contributed to its development.

It is very advantageous for everyone to learn pranic healing, especially for parents, since it is very fast and effective in healing simple and severe ailments like headaches, toothaches, fevers, sore throats, bumps, mumps, gas pain, arthritis, lung infections, heart problems, hearing problems and others.

THE
BASICS

Then the Lord God formed man out of the dust of the ground and breathed into his nostrils the breath of life, and man became a living being.

—Genesis 2:7

We get most of our ki or vital energy from the air we breathe. Every living thing depends upon breathing and cessation of breathing is cessation of life itself. From the first cry of an infant to the last gasp of the dying, there is nothing but a series of breaths. We constantly drain our life force or ki by our every thought, every act of will or motion of muscles. In consequence, constant replenishment is necessary, which is possible through breathing and other healthful practices.

—Rolando A. Carbonell

The Nature of Pranic Healing

PRANIC HEALING is based on the overall structure of the human body. The physical body is actually composed of two parts: the *visible physical body*, and the unseen or invisible energy body called the *bioplasmic body*. The visible physical body is that part of the human body that we see, touch, and are most acquainted with. The bioplasmic body is that invisible luminous energy body which interpenetrates the visible physical body and extends beyond it by four or five inches. Traditionally, clairvoyants call this energy body the *etheric body* or *etheric double*.

Pranic healing is an ancient science and art of healing that utilizes *prana* or *ki* or *vital energy* to heal the whole physical body. See figure 1 on page 4. It also involves the manipulation of ki and bioplasmic matter of the patient's body. It has also been invariably called psychic healing, magnetic healing, faith healing, ki healing, vitalic healing, and the laying on of hands.

PRANA OR KI

Prana or ki is that *vital energy* or *life force* which *keeps the body alive and healthy*. In Greek, it is called *pneuma*, in Polynesian, *mana*, and in Hebrew,

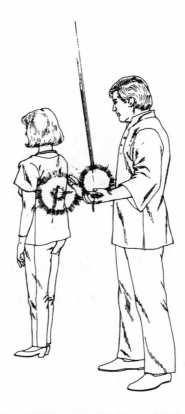

Figure 1. Pranic healing involves the transference of vital energy (ki or prana) to the patient.

ruah, which means "breath of life." The healer projects prana or vital energy or the breath of life to the patient; thereby, healing the patient. It is through this process that so called miraculous healing is accomplished.

Basically, there are three major sources of prana: solar prana, air prana, and ground prana. Solar prana is prana from sunlight. It invigorates the whole body and promotes good health. Solar prana can be obtained by exposure to sunlight or sunbathing and by drinking water that has been exposed to sunlight. Prolonged exposure or too much solar prana will harm the whole physical body since it is quite potent.

Prana contained in the air is called air prana or *air vitality globule*. Air prana is absorbed by the lungs through breathing and is also absorbed directly by the energy centers of the bioplasmic body. These energy centers are called *chakras*. More air prana can be absorbed by deep slow rhythmic breathing than by short shallow breathing. It can also be absorbed through the pores of the skin by people who have undergone certain training.

Prana contained in the ground is called ground prana or *ground vitality globule*. This is absorbed through the soles of the feet. This is done automatically and unconsciously. Walking barefooted increases the amount of ground prana absorbed by the body. One can learn to consciously draw in more ground prana to increase vitality, capacity to do more work, and ability to think more clearly.

Water absorbs prana from sunlight, air and the ground. Plants and trees absorb prana from sunlight, air, water, and ground. People and animals obtain prana from sunlight, air, ground, water, and food (fresh food contains more prana than preserved food).

Prana can also be projected to another person for healing. People with a lot of excess prana tend to make those around them feel better and livelier. However, people who are depleted tend to unconsciously absorb prana from others. This is why you may have encountered people who tend to make you feel tired or drained for no apparent reason.

Certain trees (such as pine trees or old and gigantic healthy trees) exude a lot of excess prana. Tired or sick people benefit much by lying down or resting underneath these trees. Better results can be obtained by verbally requesting the being of the tree to help the sick person get well. Anyone can learn to consciously absorb prana from these trees through the palms, so that the body would tingle and become numb due to the tremendous amount of prana absorbed. This skill can be acquired after only a few sessions of practice.

Certain areas or places tend to have more prana than others. Some of these highly energized areas tend to become healing centers.

During bad weather conditions, many people get sick, not only because of the changes in temperature, but also because of the decrease in solar and air prana (vital energy). Thus, a lot of people feel mentally and physically sluggish or become susceptible to infectious diseases. This can be counteracted by consciously absorbing prana or ki from the air and the ground. It is clairvoyantly observed that there is more prana during daytime than at night. Prana drops to a very low level at about three or four in the morning.

BIOPLASMIC BODY

Clairvoyants, with the use of their psychic faculties, have observed that every person is surrounded and interpenetrated by a luminous energy body called the bioplasmic body. Just like the visible physical body, it has a head, two eyes, two arms, etc. In other words, the bioplasmic body looks like the visible physical body. This is why clairvoyants call it the etheric double or etheric body.

The word bioplasmic comes from *bio* which means *life* and *plasma* which is the *fourth state of matter*, the first three being solid, liquid, and gas. Plasma is ionized gas or gas with positive and negative charged particles. This is not the same as blood plasma. Bioplasmic body means a living energy body made up of invisible subtle matter or etheric matter. Science, with the use of kirlian photography, has rediscovered the bioplasmic body. With the aid of kirlian photography, scientists have been able to study, observe, and take pictures of small bioplasmic articles like bioplasmic fingers, leaves, etc. It is through the bioplasmic body that prana or vital energy is absorbed and distributed throughout the whole physical body.

MERIDIANS OR BIOPLASMIC CHANNELS

Just as the visible physical body has blood vessels through which the blood flows, the bioplasmic body has fine invisible bioplasmic channels or meridians through which ki and bioplasmic matter flow to be distributed all over the body. There are several major bioplasmic *channels* and thousands of minor ones. In yoga, they call these the major and minor *nadis*. Through these channels flow prana or ki that nourishes and invigorates the whole body.

PRANA OR KI USED IN ACUPUNCTURE, ACUPRESSURE, AND REFLEXOLOGY

Acupuncture is an ancient Chinese form of medicine which uses needles to manipulate the vital energy within the patient's body; thereby, curing the patient's ailment. This is accomplished by using needles to redistribute excess prana or ki in the patient's body to the afflicted part. Congested prana in the diseased part is redistributed to other parts of the body. Blocked meridians or bioplasmic channels are cleansed or opened by directing ki to the blocked meridian.

In acupressure or in reflexology, the principle is the same as in acupuncture, except that the healer intentionally or unintentionally uses his or her own excess prana. This excess prana is directed toward the acupressure point which then goes to the meridian or bioplasmic channel and then to the afflicted part. Some acupuncturists use and direct their own ki or vital energy to the needle in order to reach the diseased part. This is done especially with patients who are very weak or depleted. I have met acupuncturists and acupressurists who are also masters of Tai Chi. They are proficient in transferring ki to their patients.

WHAT CAN PRANIC HEALING DO?

1) It can help parents bring down the temperature of their children suffering from high fever in just a few hours and heal it in a day or two in most cases.

2) It can relieve headaches, gas pains, toothaches, and muscle pains almost immediately in most cases.

3) Cough and cold can usually be cured in a day or two. Loose bowel movements can be healed in a few hours in most cases.

4) Major illnesses, such as eye, liver, kidney, and heart problems can be relieved in a few sessions and healed in a few months in many cases.

5) It increases the rate of healing by three times or more than the normal rate of healing.

All of these assume that the healer has attained a certain degree of proficiency. Any healthy person with average intelligence, an average ability to concentrate, an open but discriminating mind, and a certain degree of persistence can learn pranic healing in a relatively short period. Pranic healing is easier than learning piano or painting. It is as easy as learning to drive. Its basic principles and techniques can be learned in a few sessions. Like driving, to achieve a certain degree of proficiency requires much practice and time.

A time will come when science will make tremendous advances, not because of better instruments for discovering and measuring things, but because a few people will have at their command great spiritual powers, which at the present are seldom used. Within a few centuries, the art of spiritual healing will be increasingly developed and universally used.

—Gustaf Stromberg
Man, Mind, and the Universe

2

Auras of the Bioplasmic Body

THE BIOPLASMIC BODY interpenetrates the visible physical body and extends beyond it by four to five inches. This invisible luminous energy field which follows the contour of the visible physical body is called the *inner aura*. (See figure 2a on page 10.) In *The Human Aura*, Kilner writes:

> The idea of a human aura, a radiating luminous cloud surrounding the body, is an ancient one. Sacred images from the early Egypt, India, Greece, and Rome used this convention before it became so popular in Christian art, and before the aura was considered an attribute of ordinary everyday mortals. . . . For centuries it has been believed that clairvoyant people could actually see an aura surrounding ordinary individuals, and this aura differed from person to person in color and character, expressing the health, emotional and spiritual attributes of the subject. The visionary Swedenborg wrote in his Spiritual Diary: There is a spiritual sphere surrounding everyone as well as a natural and corporeal one.[2]

---

[2]W. J. Kilner, *The Human Aura* (York Beach, ME: Samuel Weiser, 1976). Now out of print.

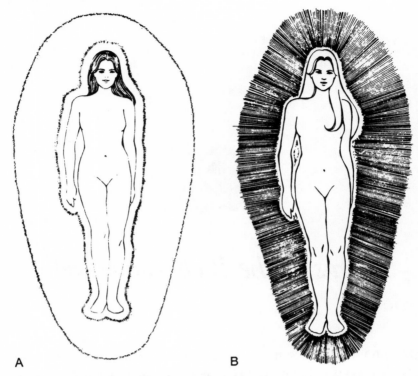

Figure 2. The outer and inner auras are shown in (A); the health aura and its health rays are shown in (B).

When the bioplasmic body becomes sick, it may be caused partially by general or localized depletion of prana in the bioplasmic body. This is called *pranic depletion*. The inner aura of the affected part is reduced to about two inches or less. For example, persons with nearsightedness usually have pranic depletion around the eye areas. The inner aura around the eye area may be smaller than two inches. However, there are cases in which an eye may suffer pranic depletion and congestion simultaneously. The more severe the sickness, the smaller is the affected inner aura. I have seen cases in which the affected inner aura had been reduced to half an inch or less. *You can learn to feel the inner auras with your palms in two to four sessions* by following the instructions in this book. Feeling the auras is called *scanning*.

Sickness may also be caused by prolonged excess prana in localized areas. This is called *pranic congestion*. The affected areas may protrude to about seven inches or more. In more severe cases, the affected inner aura may protrude to two-and-a-half feet or more. For instance, a person suffering from heart enlargement has pranic congestion around the heart, left shoulder, and upper left arm. The affected areas may protrude to about one foot in thickness.

In pranic depletion and congestion, the surrounding fine meridians or bioplasmic channels are *partially* or *severely blocked*. This means prana cannot flow freely in and out around the affected area. Clairvoyantly, these affected areas are seen as light to dark gray in color. If the affected areas are inflamed, then they appear as muddy red; with some cancer cases, they appear as muddy yellow; with appendicitis, as muddy green; and with some cases of ear problems, as muddy orange.

The bioplasmic rays project perpendicularly from the surface of the physical body. These rays are called *health rays* and they interpenetrate the inner aura. The sum of these health rays is called the *health aura*. (See figure 2b.) The health aura follows the contour of the visible physical body

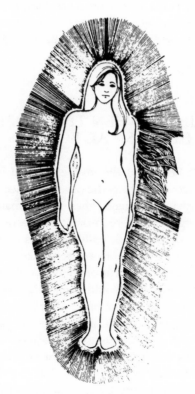

Figure 3. Drooping and entangled health rays of a sick person.

and functions as a protective force field that shields the whole body from germs and diseased bioplasmic matter in the surroundings. Toxins, wastes, germs, and diseased bioplasmic matter are expelled by the health rays predominantly through the pores. If a person is weakened, the health rays droop and are partially entangled. (See figure 3 on page 11.) Then the whole body becomes susceptible to infection. The capacity of the health rays to expel toxins, wastes, germs, and diseased bioplasmic matter is also greatly diminished. Healing is facilitated by strengthening and disentangling the health rays.

Beyond the health aura is another luminous energy field called the *outer aura*. (See figure 2a.) It interpenetrates the inner and health auras and usually extends about three feet away from the visible physical body. It is usually multicolored and shaped like an inverted egg. Its colors are influenced by the physical, emotional, and mental states of the person. Clairvoyantly, it is observed that some sick people have holes in their outer auras through which prana leaks out. Therefore, the outer aura can be considered as a force field which contains or prevents the leaking out of pranic energy. In a sense, it acts as a container or bottle for the subtle energies.

RELATIONSHIP BETWEEN THE BIOPLASMIC BODY AND THE PHYSICAL BODY

Both the bioplasmic body and the visible physical body are so closely related that what affects one affects the other and vice versa. For instance, if the bioplasmic throat is weakened then it may manifest on the visible physical body as a cough, cold, sore throat, tonsilitis or other throat related problems. Should a person accidentally slash his or her skin, there is a corresponding pranic leak in the area where there is bleeding. Initially, the affected area where there is a cut or sprain would become temporarily brighter due to pranic leak but would inevitably become grayish due to pranic depletion. If any part of the bioplasmic body is weakened due to either pranic congestion or depletion, the visible physical counterpart would either malfunction or become susceptible to infection. For example, a depleted solar plexus and liver may manifest as jaundice or hepatitis.

From these examples, it becomes quite clear that the bioplasmic body and the visible physical body affect each other. By healing the bioplasmic body, the visible physical body gets healed in the process. By regularly cleansing and energizing with prana, nearsighted eyes gradually improve and heal. A person with heart enlargement can be relieved in one or two sessions by simply decongesting the affected heart, shoulder, and upper left arm areas. Complete cure would take at least several months. By decongesting and energizing the head area, headaches can be removed in a few minutes.

Through clairvoyant observation, disease can be seen in the bioplasmic body even before it manifests itself on the visible physical body. Non-clairvoyants may scan or feel that the inner aura of the affected part is either smaller or bigger than usual. For instance, before a person suffers from colds and cough, the bioplasmic throat and lungs are pranically depleted and can be clairvoyantly observed as grayish. These areas, when scanned, can be felt as hollows in the inner aura. A person who is about to suffer from jaundice can be clairvoyantly observed as having grayishness over the solar plexus and the liver areas. Physical tests or diagnosis will show the patient as normal or healthy. Unless the patient is treated, the disease will inevitably manifest on the visible physical body.

For example, I had a patient who was a habitual drinker. Based on scanning, his solar plexus chakra (energy center) was depleted, a part of the liver was depleted and a part of the liver was congested. I told the patient that he had a liver problem and that it should be treated as soon as possible. The patient had a blood test and the medical finding showed that his liver was all right. As a result, he was hesitant to be treated. After several months, the patient suffered severe pain in the liver area and the medical finding showed that he had hepatitis. The disease must be treated before it manifests on the visible physical body. The emphasis is on pre-vention. It is a lot easier and faster to heal the disease when it is still in the bioplasmic body and has not yet manifested on the visible physical body. Manifestation of the disease can also be prevented by taking proper medication. In cases where the disease has manifested, healing should be applied as early as possible. The earlier pranic healing is applied, the faster is the rate of healing. Healing becomes more difficult if the disease has fully developed since it takes more time and more pranic energy. It is important that the disease must be treated as early as possible to ensure speedy recovery.

CHAKRAS OR ENERGY CENTERS

Chakras, or whirling energy centers, are very important parts of the bio-plasmic body. Just as the visible physical body has vital and minor organs, the bioplasmic body has major, minor, and mini chakras. Major chakras are whirling energy centers which are about three to four inches in diameter. They control and energize the major and vital organs of the visible physical body. Major chakras are just like power stations that supply vital energy to major and vital organs. When the power stations malfunction, the vital organs become sick or diseased because they do not have enough vital energy to operate properly! Minor chakras are about one to two inches in diameter. Mini chakras are smaller than one inch in diameter. Minor and mini chakras control and energize the less important parts of the visible physical body. The chakras interpenetrate and extend beyond the visible physical body. They have several important functions as follows:

1) They absorb, digest, and distribute prana to the different parts of the body.

2) The chakras control, energize, and are responsible for the proper functioning of the whole physical body and its different parts and organs. The endocrine glands are controlled and energized by some of the major chakras. The endocrine glands can be stimulated or inhibited by controlling or manipulating the major chakras. A lot of ailments are caused partially by malfunctioning of the chakras.

3) Some chakras are sites or centers of the psychic faculties. Activation of certain chakras (energy centers) may result in the development of certain psychic faculties. For example, one of the easiest and safest chakras to activate are the hand chakras. These are located at the center of the palms. By activating the hand chakras, one develops the ability to feel subtle energies and the ability to feel the outer, health, and inner auras. This can simply be accomplished by regularly concentrating on them. In this book, it is called sensitizing the hands.

We will discuss the basic chakras in more depth in the next chapter.

PSYCHOSOMATIC DISEASES

Uncontrolled emotions, inhibitions, and suppressed feelings such as anger, intense worry, prolonged irritation, inhibitions or suppressed emotions, and frustrations have undesirable potent effects on the bioplasmic body. For instance, anger and frustration results in pranic depletion around the solar plexus and abdominal areas or may manifest as pranic congestion around the solar plexus and heart area. In the first case, it manifests itself as indigestion or loose bowel movements. In the long run, it may manifest itself as ulcers or as a gall bladder problem. In the second case, it may manifest itself as a heart enlargement or other heart related problems. It seems that a certain type of negative emotion may manifest as a certain type of disease in one patient but may manifest as another type of disease in another.

Anger and intense worry devitalize the whole bioplasmic body so that the body becomes susceptible to all kinds of diseases. Negative emotions cause disturbances in the bioplasmic body so that the whole physical body becomes sick. You may have experienced that after an intense anger or an intense altercation, you felt physically exhausted or became sick. This is because both the bioplasmic and visible physical bodies are drained of prana and became susceptible to infection.

If the ailment is of emotional origin, the healer must not only give pranic healing but also psychological counselling. The patient should be asked to undergo a course in character building and to meditate regularly to help overcome these negative emotional tendencies. Through daily inner reflection and meditation, the patient would develop greater self-awareness and emotional maturity. These would greatly improve the ability to control and channel emotions, thus, vastly improving health. It should be noted that in this case, pranic healing will not produce a permanent cure unless there is a corresponding emotional change. It is like extinguishing a fire caused by an arsonist without bothering to catch the culprit. What is to prevent the arsonist from burning the house again once it has been rebuilt? The root cause of the disease must be removed so that permanent healing can take place.

MIND INFLUENCE ON THE BIOPLASMIC BODY

Clairvoyants have observed that the visible physical body is patterned or molded after the bioplasmic body. The mind can intentionally or unintentionally influence the pattern of the bioplasmic body. Men well-versed in esoteric studies encourage their pregnant wives to look at beautiful things, to listen to harmonious music, to feel and think positively, to engage in serious studies, and to avoid the opposites. These activities affect not only the features of the unborn baby but also the emotional and mental potentialities and tendencies. If the influences are positive, then the effects are positive. If the influences are negative, then the effects are negative. Pregnant women should take note of this so they will be able to bear better children.

This idea that the mind can influence and actually mold the bioplasmic body to a certain degree is not new. There is a biblical story in Genesis that illustrates this point. This concerns the manner in which Jacob was able to successfully build up his own flock. Jacob had been working for his father-in-law, Laban, for approximately twenty years and yearned to establish himself financially. An agreement was made between Laban and Jacob that all goats born speckled, spotted, and striped and all lambs born black would belong to Jacob. Laban, being a shrewd businessman, that same day removed all the male goats that were streaked or spotted, and all the speckled or spotted female goats (all that had white on them), including all the dark-colored lambs. Genetically, it would be unlikely, if not very difficult, to breed the types of goats and lambs promised to Jacob.

Jacob, through the guidance of the Lord, "took fresh-cut branches from poplar, almond and plane trees and made white stripes on them by peeling the bark and exposing the white inner wood of the branches. Then he placed the peeled branches in all the watering troughs, so that they would be directly in front of the flocks when they came to drink. When the flocks were in heat and came to drink, they mated in front of the branches. And they bore young that were streaked or speckled or spotted" (Genesis 30:37–39). In this way, Jacob became very prosperous.

From this story, it becomes clear that what we see, feel, and think can influence the bioplasmic body, especially that of the unborn baby.

EXTERNAL AND INTERNAL FACTORS OF DISEASES

In the understanding of diseases, one should take into consideration the external and internal factors or the seen and unseen causes. External factors mean those physical factors which contribute to disease like germs, malnutrition, toxins, pollutants, lack of exercise, poor breathing habits, insufficient water intake, etc. Internal factors mean the emotional and bioplasmic factors which contribute to diseases, such as negative emotions, blocked meridians, pranic depletion and congestion, chakral malfunctioning, etc.

For instance, an emotional factor may lead to the weakening of the solar plexus chakra (a major energy center located at the solar plexus) and of the liver, plus an attack from the hepatitis virus or from toxins (such as carbon tetrachloride or phosphorus) will lead to a severe inflammation of the liver. The external factor is the virus or the toxin. The internal factors are the negative emotions and weakening of the solar plexus chakra and the liver that makes the liver vulnerable to viral infection.

If the solar plexus chakra and liver are in good condition, and if the person is of higher vitality, then the probability of contracting the disease is decreased. The body's defense mechanism or detoxifying and eliminating system would likely overcome the virus or the toxin.

The application of pranic healing would cleanse, strengthen, and gradually restore the solar plexus chakra and the liver to their normal conditions. This can be done with or without the aid of drugs.

Diseases may manifest under the following conditions:

1) Due to the presence of external and internal factors.

2) Due to the presence of an overwhelming internal factor only. For example, a person harboring intense anger and frustration may cause severe pranic congestion around the solar plexus chakra, and heart chakra in the long run. Even if this person were to watch his or her diet, he or she would still end up with a heart problem like heart enlargement. Another example: habitual tension or stress may result in pranic congestion around the eye area and, in the long run, may result in glaucoma. (Note: Not all glaucomae are of emotional origin.)

3) Due to the presence of an overwhelming external factor only. For instance, taking a large dose of poison would certainly be fatal even if your bioplasmic body were in perfect condition. Or, for example, poor reading habits would eventually result in eye defects.

THE FUNCTIONS OF THE BIOPLASMIC BODY

1) It absorbs, distributes, and energizes the whole physical body with prana or ki. Prana or ki is that vital energy or life force which nourishes the whole body so that it could, together with its different organs, function properly and normally. Without prana, the body would die.

2) It acts as a mold or pattern for the visible physical body. This allows the visible physical body to maintain its shape, form and feature despite years of continuous metabolism. To be more exact, the visible physical body is molded after the bioplasmic body. If the bioplasmic body is de-

fective, then the visible physical body is defective. They are so closely related that what affects one affects the other. If one gets sick, the other also gets sick. If one gets healed, the other also gets healed. This may manifest gradually or almost instantaneously, assuming that there are no interfering factors.

3) The bioplasmic body, through the chakras or whirlng energy centers, controls and is responsible for the proper functioning of the whole physical body and its different parts and organs. This includes the endocrine glands. The endocrine glands are external manifestations of some of the major chakras. A lot of sicknesses are caused partially by the malfunctioning of one or more chakras.

4) The bioplasmic body, through its health rays and health auras, serves as a protective shield against germs and diseased bioplasmic matter. Toxins, wastes, and germs are *expelled* by the health rays predominantly via the pores; thereby, purifying the whole physical body.

BASIC PROBLEMS AND TREATMENTS IN PRANIC HEALING

Pranic or bioplasmic healing involves the use of prana and the manipulation of bioplasmic matter of the patient's body. The following are the basic problems and treatments encountered in pranic healing:

1) In areas where there is pranic depletion, cleansing and pranic energizing are applied to the affected areas. The emphasis is on energizing.

2) In areas where there is pranic congestion, diseased congested bioplasmic matter is removed or extracted from the affected areas. This is followed by projecting prana to the treated area. The emphasis is on cleansing or decongesting.

3) A malfunctioning chakra is restored by simply cleansing and energizing it with prana.

4) Drooping and entangled health rays are disentangled and strengthened.

5) Blocked meridians or bioplasmic channels are cleansed and energized.

6) Prana leaking out through holes in the outer aura are sealed.

7) Specific types of prana are applied to produce specific results. Certain illnesses need specific type or types of prana to produce faster results.

COURSE OUTLINE

We will study four levels of pranic healing, moving from simple to more complicated concepts, and from easy to difficult techniques. As you study the material make sure you are comfortable with the first level before moving to the next.

Level One: *Elementary Pranic Healing*: At this level, the concepts and techniques are easy to learn. Tactile concentration is required. It takes about three to five sessions to learn the basic principles and techniques and to be able to do simple pranic healing. About one to two months of regular practice and application are necessary to become proficient.

Level Two: *Intermediate Pranic Healing*: This level is still easy. Pranic breathing is used at this level. The major chakras are explained fully. Visual concentration is still not required. It takes about three to five sessions to learn the basic principles and techniques to be able to start healing more difficult cases. To become proficient, it takes about two months of regular practice and application.

Level Three: *Distant Pranic Healing*: This level involves a gradual development of one's psychic faculty. It may take at least several months to several years of regular practice and application to become very accurate in diagnosis and to produce specific accurate predetermined results.

Level Four: *Advanced Pranic Healing*: Visualization is definitely required. A more thorough knowledge of the nature of disease and the properties of the different types of prana is required.

REFERENCES AND RECOMMENDED READING

There are several books you should read to help you with your study: *The Etheric Double* by A. E. Powell. (The Theosophical Publishing House, Quest Books. Wheaton, IL, 1969.) Essentially, this book is a treatise on the etheric body and etheric phenomena. Its contents are largely based on the writings of Madame Blavatsky, C. W. Leadbeater, and Annie Besant. These highly developed clairvoyants conducted clairvoyant researches and experiments. They recorded their observations and conclusions in their writings from 1897–1923.

The following is a summation of main points relevant to the study of pranic healing that are discussed in this book:

1) The whole physical body is actually composed of two bodies: the visible physical body and the invisible etheric body which is made up of finer substances called etheric matter. This etheric body corresponds to what is now called the bioplasmic body.

2) The etheric body is the vehicle of prana or ki.

3) The etheric body has many nadis or etheric channels through which prana or ki flows. These etheric channels are the equivalent of the meridians or bioplasmic channels.

4) The etheric body is the mold or pattern of the visible physical body.

5) The etheric body has several chakras or etheric whirling centers which absorb, digest, and distribute prana and is responsible for the proper functioning of the whole body.

6) Some chakras are psychic faculty centers or the sites of our psychic faculties.

7) Prana can be obtained from sunlight, air, and trees.

8) The visible physical body and its etheric body are so closely inter-related that what affects one also affects the other. Healing is brought about by removing the diseased etheric matter from the patient's etheric body and by transferring or projecting prana from the healer's etheric body to that of the patient's etheric body.

9) A strong health aura acts as a protective shield against germs and infection.

10) People whose limbs have been amputated sometimes complain that they still feel the limb in place. The reason for this is that the etheric counterpart or the etheric mold is still intact.

It should be noted that the existence of the etheric body and other important points mentioned in the preceding items were later verified or rediscovered by Russian scientists. Students should also read *Psychic Discoveries Behind the Iron Curtain* by Sheila Ostrander and Lynn Schroeder (Englewood Cliffs N.J.: Prentice Hall, 1970. Bantam edition 1971). This book describes the extensive scientific investigations on psychic phenomena being conducted in the Soviet Union. Many of the findings merely reconfirm what has been known by esoteric students since the ancient times. All references are made to the Bantam edition. The following is a summation of points students should consider:

1) In 1939, Semyon Davidovich Kirlian and his wife developed kirlian photography based on a high frequency electric field which is used to take pictures of a portion of the invisible energy body or the bioplasmic body (Chap. 16, pp. 202–206).

2) Based on the studies of the Kirlians, it has been observed that disease first manifests on the bioplasmic body before it appears on the visible physical body (Chap. 16, pp. 207–210).

3) At the highly respected Kirov State University in Alma-Ata, a group of biologists, biochemists and biophysicists declared that the bioplasmic body is not merely some sort of plasma-like constellation of ionized, excited electrons, protons and possibly some other particle, but is a whole unified organism in itself which acts as a unit that gives off its own electromagnetic fields (Chap. 17, p. 217).

4) Emotions, states of mind, and thoughts affect the bioplasmic body (Chap. 16, p. 209).

5) Based on the findings of the State University of Kazakhstan, the energy body has a specific organizing pattern that determines the form of the organism. For instance, Dr. Alexander Studitsky at the Institute of Animal Morphology in Moscow minced up muscle tissue and packed it into a wound in a rat's body. An entirely new muscle was grown. From this they concluded that there is some sort of organizing pattern (Chap. 17, p. 218).

6) If a person loses a finger or an arm, he or she still retains the bioplasmic finger or arm so that sometimes he or she feels that it is still there (Chap. 17, p. 216).

7) Dr. Mikhail Kuzmich Gaikin, a Leningrad scientist, confirmed the existence of bioplasmic channels and centers that correspond to the meridians and the acupuncture points described in the ancient Chinese medicine (Chap. 18, pp. 226–229). With the aid of the tobiscope, he accurately pinpointed the location of the acupuncture points. Later, a young physicist, Victor Adamenko, invented an improved version of the tobiscope and called it the CCAP—Conductivity of the Channels of Acupuncture Points which not only locates acupuncture points but also numerically graphs reactions and changes in the bioplasmic body (Chap. 18, p. 232).

8) The acupuncture points correspond to the bright spots in the bioplasmic body (Chap. 18, p. 226).

9) The Russians also seriously considered the possibility of stimulating certain points in the bioplasmic body to activate latent psychic abilities (Chap. 18, pp. 231–233).

10) Researches done on Russian psychic healers indicate that psychic healing involves a transfer of energy from the bioplasmic body of the healer to the bioplasmic body of his patient (Chap. 18, p. 224).

The Chakras by C. W. Leadbeater (The Theosophical Publishing House, Adyar, Madras, 1927) is another book that deals with the different types of prana once air prana has been digested by the chakras. It also discusses the negative effects of alcohol, drugs, and tobacco on the etheric body. It contains ten colored illustrations of the chakras based on the clairvoyant observations of Mr. Leadbeater.

Theories of the Chakras: Bridge to Higher Consciousness by Hiroshi Motoyama (The Theosophical Publishing House, Wheaton, IL, 1981) contains a discussion of the scientific experiments and personal experience of Dr. Hiroshi Motoyama on the chakras. It also gives instructions on how to activate the chakras. The Chinese acupuncture meridians are compared with the Indian nadis. This book is quite interesting and very informative.

You should also read *Esoteric Healing* by Alice Bailey (Lucis Publishing Company. NY, 1953) and *The Aura* by W. J. Kilner, 1911. This book was published by Samuel Weiser, Inc. (York Beach, ME, 1976) but it is now out of print. You may be able to find a copy in a second hand bookshop.

LEVEL ONE: ELEMENTARY PRANIC HEALING

When the body is worn out and the blood is exhausted [of its vital energy] is it still possible to achieve good results?

No, because there is no more energy left . . . vitality and energy are considered the foundation of life . . . and how then can a disease be cured when there is no vital energy left within the body?

The Yellow Emperor's
Classic of Internal Medicine
(Huang Ti Nei Ching Su Wen)

And Jesus said, . . . someone has touched me, for I know that power has gone out of me. . . . she said in the presence of all the people for what purpose she had touched him and how she was healed immediately.

Luke 8:45–47

3

Cleansing and Energizing

IN PRANIC HEALING, there are two basic principles: cleansing and energizing the patient's bioplasmic body with prana or vital energy. It is by cleansing or removing the diseased bioplasmic matter from the affected chakra and the diseased organ, and by energizing them with sufficient prana or vital energy, that healing is accomplished. These two basic principles are the very foundation of pranic healing. (See figure 4.)

The basic principle of cleansing and energizing is clearly manifested in the body because the body is cleansed by exhaling used-up air or carbon dioxide, and is energized by inhaling fresh air or oxygen. The physical body cleanses itself through its eliminative system, and is energized through proper food. The healer must give equal emphasis to cleansing as well as energizing the bioplasmic body.

Cleansing is necessary to remove the devitalized diseased bioplasmic matter in the whole body or in the affected part or parts, and to clear up blocked bioplasmic channels. The health rays are cleansed, combed, and strengthened.

It must be noted that the affected part should be thoroughly cleansed before and/or after energizing is done. For more severe cases, the entire bioplasmic body has to be cleansed. Very often, after initial cleansing, the patient should be partially energized to facilitate further cleansing. This is

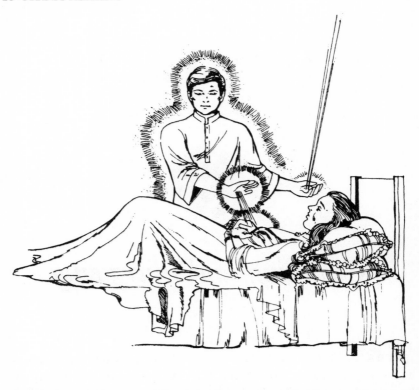

Figure 4. Pranic healing is accomplished by removing the diseased energy and by energizing the affected parts with prana or vital energy.

like first sweeping a very dirty floor and then adding soap and water or cleansing chemical to clean and remove the stubborn dirt. The whole process may be repeated over and over again until the bioplasmic body is normalized. Without cleansing, the patient may suffer a radical reaction. Radical reaction means the drastic steps the body takes in order to correct and normalize its condition. This is usually painful and uncomfortable, and may appear as an initial worsening condition. However, the body gradually improves after this radical reaction. This radical reaction is quite unnecessary and can be avoided.

One such case is that of a patient who suffered from chronic abdominal pain, loose bowel movements and vomiting due to emotional factors. There was pranic congestion around her abdominal area. Energizing with prana was applied without cleansing the affected part. Although she was relieved, within twenty to thirty minutes the pain, loose bowel movements and vomiting recurred and intensified. These were radical reactions or steps taken by the whole physical body to cleanse and remove the diseased congested bioplasmic matter from itself and to normalize its condition. Three hours later, cleansing and energizing with prana was applied to her abdominal area and she was completely relieved and cured.

Cleansing is necessary to facilitate the absorption of prana or ki by the affected part. This is similar to pouring fresh coffee into a cup that is already filled with stale coffee, or trying to replace the dirty water inside a sponge by pouring clean water on top of it. This approach is slow and quite wasteful. Fresh prana cannot flow easily into the affected part since the affected part is filled with diseased bioplasmic matter and the bioplasmic channels are blocked. The projected fresh prana is also not fully absorbed by the treated part and because of this there is a strong possibility that the ailment would recur immediately or within a short period of time.

There are several reasons why cleansing should be done before energizing:

1) Cleansing is necessary to facilitate the absorption of prana or ki.

2) Healing takes a longer time without cleansing and more prana is required to heal the patient.

3) A possible radical reaction could be induced if cleansing is not done before or after energizing.

4) Cleansing is necessary to reduce the risk of damaging the finer bioplasmic channels (called meridians or energy centers).

In simple cases, cleansing the bioplasmic body and/or the affected part is usually sufficient to heal the patient. In other cases, the diseased bioplasmic part is so depleted that the healer has to facilitate the healing process by energizing with prana.

HAND AND FINGER CHAKRAS

There are two very important chakras located at the center of each palm. These chakras are called the left hand chakra and right hand chakra. (See figure 5 on page 28). They are usually about one inch in diameter. Some pranic healers have hand chakras as big as two inches or more in diameter. Although the hand chakras are considered as minor chakras, they have

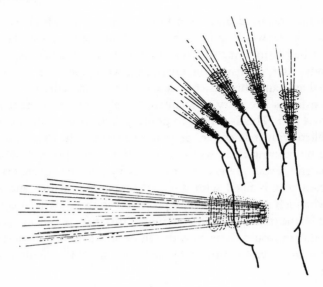

Figure 5. Hand and finger chakras.

very important functions in pranic healing. It is through the hand chakras that prana is absorbed from the surroundings and projected to the patient. Both the right and left hand chakras are capable of absorbing and projecting prana or ki. But for right-handed persons, it is easier to absorb through the left hand chakra and project through the right hand chakra and vice versa for left-handed people.

There is a mini chakra in each finger. These chakras are also capable of absorbing and projecting prana. The hand chakras project less concentrated or gentler prana while the finger chakras project more intense or stronger prana. With infants, the aged, and very weak patients, it is advisable to energize them slowly and gently by using the hand chakras.

By stimulating or activating the hand chakras, the hands become sensitized; thereby developing the ability to feel subtler matter and to scan the different auras. It is through scanning that the healer can locate the diseased areas in the bioplasmic body.

FIVE BASIC TECHNIQUES

There are basic techniques you will need to learn in order to work with pranic healing. They are:

1) Sensitizing the hands;

2) Scanning the inner aura;

3) Sweeping or cleansing (general and localized);

4) Energizing with prana (Hand Chakras Technique) to draw in prana and to project prana;

5) Stabilizing the projected prana.

All these techniques have been tried and tested. Most of you will be able to produce positive results in just a few sessions by properly following the instructions. It is very important to maintain an open mind and to be persevering. Practice immediately what you have read and try the techniques for at least four sessions.

SENSITIZING THE HANDS

Since it would take a considerable amount of time to develop the auric sight, you should try to sensitize your hands in order to feel the bioplasmic energy field or the inner aura in order to determine which areas of the patient's bioplasmic body are depleted or congested.

1) Place your hands about three inches apart facing each other. Do not tense, just relax. (See figure 6.)

2) Concentrate on feeling the center of your palms and simultaneously be aware of your entire hand for about five to ten minutes. At the same time, inhale and exhale slowly and rhythmically. Concentration is facilitated by pressing the centers of your palms with your thumbs before starting. It is by concentrating at the center of the palms that the hand chakras are activated, thereby sensitizing the hands or enabling the hands to feel subtle energy or matter.

Eighty to ninety percent of you will be able to feel a tingling sensation, heat, pressure or rhythmic pulsation between the palms on the first try. It is important to feel the pressure or the rhythmic pulsation.

3) Proceed immediately to scanning after sensitizing your hands.

4) Practice sensitizing your hands for at least two weeks. Your hands should be more or less permanently sensitized after two weeks of practice.

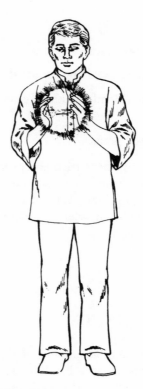

Figure 6. Sensitizing the hands.

5) Do not be discouraged if you do not feel anything on the first try. Continue your practice, you should be able to feel these subtle sensations on the third or fourth session. It is very important to keep an open mind and to concentrate properly.

SCANNING

In scanning, it is helpful (but not really necessary) to first learn how to feel the size and shape of the outer and health auras before scanning the inner aura. This is to make your hands more sensitive since both the outer and health auras are subtler than the inner aura and also to prove to yourself the existence of the outer and health auras. In healing, we are primarily interested in scanning the inner aura. It is in scanning the inner aura that the trouble spots can be located.

When scanning with your hands, always concentrate at the center of your palms. It is by concentrating at the center of your palms that the hand chakras remain or are further activated; thereby making the hands sensitive to subtle energy or matter. Without doing this you will have difficulty in scanning.

Scanning the Outer Aura

1) Stand about twelve feet away from the subject with your palms facing the subject and your arms slightly outstretched.

2) Slowly walk toward the subject, simultaneously trying to feel with your sensitized hands the subject's outer aura. Concentrate at the center of your palms when scanning.

3) Stop when you feel heat, a tingling sensation or a slight pressure. You are now feeling the outer aura. Try feeling the size and shape of the outer aura, its width from head to waist, waist to feet, and from front to back. In most cases, it will feel like an inverted egg; the top being wider than the bottom.

4) It is very important that you gradually learn to feel the aura in terms of pressure in order to be more accurate in determining the width of the outer, health, and inner auras.

5) The outer aura is usually about three feet in radius but in some cases it may be more than six feet wide. Some hyperactive children have outer auras as big as nine feet.

Scanning the Health Aura

1) After determining the size and shape of the outer aura, gradually move forward a little, still retaining the earlier position.

2) Stop when you feel the subtle sensations again. These sensations may be slightly more intense. You are now feeling the health aura. Feel the size and shape of the health aura.

The health aura is usually about two feet in width. When someone is sick, his or her health rays droop and are entangled and the health aura decreases in size. Sometimes, the health aura may decrease to twelve inches or less. The health aura of a very healthy and energetic person may be as big as three feet or more. It usually feels like a tapering cylinder, bigger at the top and smaller at the bottom.

Scanning the Inner Aura

1) Proceed to feel the inner aura with one or both hands. Move your hands slowly and slightly back and forth to feel the inner aura. The inner aura is usually about five inches in thickness. Concentrate at the center of your palms when scanning. It is by concentrating at the center of the palms that your hand chakras remain or are further activated; thereby making your hands sensitive to subtle energy or matter.

2) Scan your subject from head to foot and from front to back. Scan the left part and right part. For example, scan the left and right ears, or scan the right and left lungs. When the inner aura of the right part and left part of the body are scanned, they should have about the same thickness. If one part is bigger or smaller than the other part, then there is something wrong with it. For instance, the ears of a patient were scanned and it was found out that the inner aura of the left ear was about five inches thick, while the inner aura of the right ear was only about two inches thick. The

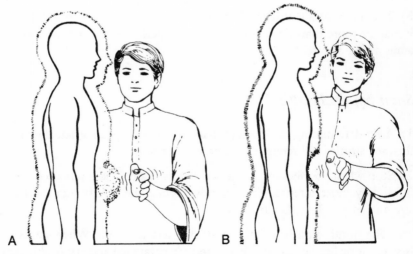

Figure 7. Scanning the inner aura. (A) shows congestion while (B) shows pranic depletion.

patient, when questioned, revealed that the right ear has been partially deaf for the past seventeen years.

3) Special attention should be given to the spine, to the vital organs, and to the major chakras. In many cases, a portion of the spine is usually either congested or depleted even if the patient does not complain about back problem.

4) In scanning the throat area, the chin should be raised upward in order to get accurate scanning. The inner aura of the chin tends to interfere or camouflage the actual condition of the throat.

5) Scanning of the lungs should be done at the back and at the sides rather than the front in order to get accurate results. The nipples have two mini chakras that tend to interfere in the proper scanning of the lungs. A more advanced technique is to scan the lungs at the front, at the back and at the sides by using two fingers, instead of using the entire hand.

6) Special attention should be given to the solar plexus since many diseases of emotional origin negatively affect the solar plexus chakra.

Interpreting Results

In scanning your patient, you will notice that there are *hollows* or *protrusions* in some areas of the patient's inner aura. When the area is hollow, this is caused by *pranic depletion*. The affected part is depleted of prana or there is insufficient prana in the affected area. The surrounding fine meridians are partially or severely blocked, preventing fresh prana from other parts to flow freely and vitalize the affected part. In pranic depletion, the affected chakra is depleted and filled with dirty diseased bioplasmic matter. And usually it is partially underactivated. (See figure 7.)

When the area is protruding, this is caused by *pranic congestion* or *bioplasmic congestion*. It means that there is too much prana and bioplasmic matter on the affected area and the surrounding fine meridians are partially or severely blocked. The excess prana and bioplasmic matter cannot flow out freely. This congested prana and bioplasmic matter becomes devitalized and diseased after a certain period of time since fresh prana cannot flow in freely, or its inflow is greatly reduced and the devitalized matter cannot flow out freely or its outflow is greatly reduced. In pranic congestion, the affected chakra is congested and filled with diseased bioplasmic matter. Usually it is partially overactivated. (See figure 7b.)

An affected part may have pranic congestion and pranic depletion simultaneously. It means a portion of the affected part is hollow and another portion is protruding. For instance, a liver is congested or protruding on the left portion and is hollow or depleted on the right portion. Another example is that a portion of the left heart is congested or protruding and a portion of the right heart is severely depleted.

The smaller the inner aura, the more severe is the pranic depletion. The bigger the protrusion of the inner aura, the more congested is the affected part. The smaller or bigger the inner aura of the diseased part, the more severe the sickness.

Students should note that an area may have a *temporary pranic surplus* in which case there is nothing wrong with it. For instance, a person who has been sitting down for a long time may have a big protrusion of the inner aura around the buttocks area when scanned. Since the surrounding meridians are not blocked, the condition normalizes after a short period of time. Or, an area may have *temporary pranic reduction*, in which case there is also nothing wrong with it. An altercation that has just occurred is likely to cause a temporary pranic reduction around the solar plexus. After a few hours of rest, the condition will normalize. Habitual altercation or anger may cause pranic depletion around the solar plexus which results in abdominal ailments and possibly heart disease.

The physical condition of the patient should be carefully observed and the patient should be thoroughly questioned or interviewed before jumping to any conclusion.

As stated earlier, diseases manifest first on the bioplasmic body before manifesting on the visible physical body. There are cases in which there is pranic depletion or pranic congestion in the inner aura of an affected part but medical examination would show a negative result or the part is normal. In this case, the disease has not yet manifested on the visible physical body. *Therefore, pranic healing should be applied to the disease before it can manifest physically.*

SWEEPING

Sweeping is generally a cleansing technique. It can also be used for energizing and distributing excess prana. When cleansing is done on the whole bioplasmic body, it is called *general sweeping*. Cleansing done on specific parts of the body is called *localized sweeping*.

The hands are used in sweeping. There are two hand positions: the *cupped-hand position* and the *spread-finger position*. These two hand positions are used alternately. The cupped-hand position is more effective in removing the diseased bioplasmic matter and the spread-finger position is more effective in combing and disentangling the health rays. General sweeping has been called aura cleansing or combing by some esoteric students.

Sweeping produces the following results:

1) It removes congested and diseased bioplasmic matter. Blocked meridians or bioplasmic channels are cleansed and unclogged. This allows prana from other parts of the body to flow to the affected part, facilitating the healing process.

2) Expelling of toxins, wastes, germs, and dirty bioplasmic matter is greatly facilitated by disentangling and partially strengthening the health rays. The health rays are further strengthened by energizing the whole body with prana.

3) By disentangling and strengthening the health rays, the health aura, which acts as a protective shield, is normalized. This increases one's resistance against infection.

4) Sweeping automatically seals holes in the outer aura through which prana leaks out. Without sealing the holes in the outer aura, the healing process is very slow even if the patient is energized with prana because prana would just simply leak out. This is one of the contributing factors in regression. The disease sometimes comes back in a few minutes or hours after the patient has been healed when this sealing is not done.

5) Absorption of prana by the patient is greatly facilitated after sweeping or cleansing.

6) Sweeping is also used to distribute excess prana in a treated area to other parts of the body after it has been energized to prevent possible congestion.

7) Sweeping is used to energize by directing excess prana from the surrounding areas of the body or from a chakra or chakras to the affected part that is low in prana. For instance, a mild form of arthritis of the fingers was cured in minutes just by cleansing the fingers and sweeping or directing the excess prana from the hand chakra to the affected fingers.

8) Radical reaction is reduced or avoided by simply sweeping the patient thoroughly.

Sweeping is a very important pranic healing technique and it is very easy to learn. It cleanses, strengthens, and greatly facilitates the healing process. Many simple illnesses can be healed just by sweeping.

General Sweeping Exercise

General sweeping is done with a series of *downward sweeping movements* only. In downward sweeping, you start from the head and work down to the feet. Upward sweeping movements are not used in cleansing but are used only to reawaken patients who may have fallen asleep or who may have become slightly drowsy. In upward sweeping, you start from the feet and work up to the head. See figure 8.

1) Cup your hands and place them six inches above the head of the patient. Do not unnecessarily touch the patient. Maintain a distance of about two inches between the patient's body and your hands.

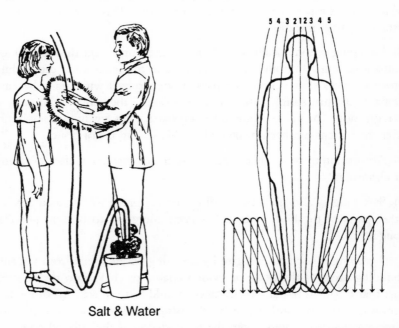

Salt & Water

Figure 8. General sweeping. By cleansing or removing the diseased energy, circulation of vital energy, or prana, is enhanced, thereby increasing the rate of healing.

2) With your hands still cupped, sweep your hands slowly downward from the head to the feet following line #1 as shown in figure 8. Slightly raise your hands and strongly flick them downward to throw away the dirty diseased bioplasmic matter. This is very important to avoid recontaminating the patient with the diseased bioplasmic matter; and also to avoid contaminating yourself, which would result not only as pain in your fingers, hands, and palms, but may result in the weakening of your body and/or illness similar to that of the patient.

3) Repeat the process discussed in procedure 2 (above) with spread-finger position instead of the cupped-hand position. This is to disentangle and strengthen the health rays. This is called combing.

4) Repeat the whole process in procedures 2 and 3 on lines 2, 3, 4, and 5 as shown in figure 8.

5) Apply downward sweeping on the back of the patient by following procedures 2, 3, and 4.

6) It is very important to concentrate and to form an intention to remove the diseased bioplasmic matter. Without this, the sweeping process becomes less effective and more time-consuming. It is the intention or the application of the will with the aid of the hands that the diseased bioplasmic matter is thoroughly and quickly removed. With regular practice, you can apply sweeping with great ease and with minimum effort.

7) After the downward sweeping, some patients may become sleepy. You may apply a few upward sweeping movements to reawaken or make the patient more alert. There is no need to flick your hands after the upward sweeping. Upward sweeping is not a cleansing technique, but a technique to reawaken the patient. It should be applied only after the patient has been relatively cleansed. Warning: Upward sweeping before applying the downward sweeping may result in the diseased bioplasmic matter going to or getting stuck in the head area, which may have negative physical effects.

Localized Sweeping Exercise

1) Place your hand or hands above the affected area and slowly sweep away the diseased bioplasmic matter. This is just like cleaning a dirty object with your hand. (See figure 9 on page 38.)

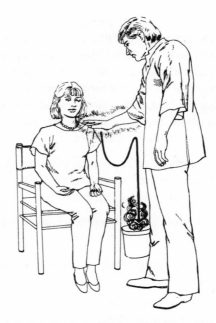

Figure 9. Localized sweeping. The rate of healing is increased by cleansing or removing the diseased energy from the affected part.

2) Strongly flick your hand to throw away the dirty bioplasmic matter.

3) The sweeping movements can be done in any direction: vertically, horizontally, diagonally or in L-shape.

Sweeping is very easy and can be learned almost immediately by most people. Sometimes in localized sweeping, the diseased bioplasmic matter is transferred from the affected part to another part of the body. For instance, one practitioner was sweeping away the congested bioplasmic matter at the back of the head of a patient, and part of it was transferred to the neck and shoulder areas. This caused the pain at the back of the head to partially move to the neck and shoulder areas. Should you encounter a similar situation, just simply apply localized sweeping on the new affected area.

How many times should general sweeping and localized sweeping be applied on a patient? The answer is as many times as required. There is no fixed number of times. Usually, I apply general sweeping once or twice and localized sweeping four or five times. However, in the case of a dog dying due to an accidental intake of slow acting poison, it was necessary to apply general sweeping and localized sweeping twenty to thirty times per session since after each sweeping and partially removing the darkish grey bioplasmic matter from the dog, the darkish grey matter would reappear after a few seconds and later after a few minutes. Sweeping and energizing was applied alternately. This whole process was repeated once every two hours and three times the first day. Healing was continued for the next few days. After about two weeks the dog became relatively active and healthy.

In case of poisoning, do not try to use only pranic healing. Get proper medical treatment and apply pranic healing to strengthen and facilitate the healing process. As stated earlier, a disease or illness could be caused by internal and/or external factors. If the cause is malnutrition, obviously enough nourishing food or nutritional supplements should be taken by the patient. Since chemical poison is a physical or external factor, then one should definitely use a physical or chemical form of treatment. Pranic healing should also be used to minimize the damage done to the body and to greatly facilitate the healing process.

In the case of the dying dog, the poison was already fully assimilated into its system and the veterinarian did not have any antidote; therefore, pranic healing was used alone because it was the only solution available at that time.

Although there are probably some great yogi, shamans or healers who can neutralize poison in their own bodies or the body of another person, who among us belongs to this caliber? In pranic healing, as well as in other field of activities, one should be fully aware of one's capabilities and limitations and should use sound judgment or common sense in making decisions.

ENERGIZING WITH PRANA: HAND CHAKRA TECHNIQUE

When projecting prana to the patient's bioplasmic body, you should simultaneously draw in air prana or air vitality globule from the surroundings. This prevents draining or exhausting yourself and becoming susceptible to infection and diseases.

There are many ways of drawing in prana and projecting prana; one of the safest and easiest ways is through the hand chakras. One of the hand chakras is used to draw in air prana and the other to project prana

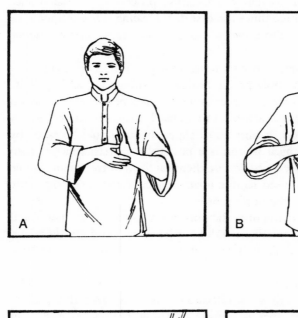
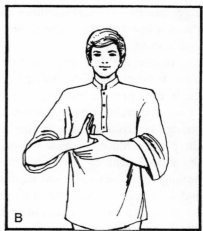
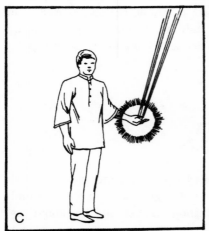
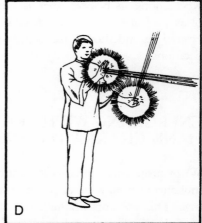

Figure 10. Energizing with prana using the hand chakra technique.

or vital energy to the patient. Both left and right hand chakras can either predominantly draw in or project prana. The hand chakra is alternately drawing in and projecting prana at a rapid rate. Whether it predominantly draws in prana or predominantly projects prana is a matter of intention or willing. You can use either the right hand chakra to project prana and the left hand chakra to draw in prana, or vice versa. This is a matter of personal preference. With right-handed people, it is easier to draw in prana using the left hand chakra and project prana with the right chakra, and vice versa for left-handed people. See figure 10.

Prana is drawn in through one of the hand chakras and projected through the other hand chakra. Attention or concentration should be focused on the hand chakras (on the centers of the palms) and on the part to be treated, with more emphasis on the hand chakras. Focusing too much on the part being treated is a mistake commonly made by beginners. This tends to reduce the flow of prana coming in and going out.

Use the following procedure:

1) Press the center of your palms with your thumb to facilitate your concentration.

2) Concentrate or focus your attention at the center of the palm that will be used for drawing in pranic energy for about ten to fifteen seconds. This is to partially activate the hand chakra, enhancing its ability to draw in pranic energy. If you intend to draw in pranic energy through your left hand, then concentrate at its center.

3) Place the other hand near the affected part and concentrate simultaneously at the centers of both hands. If you intend to project with your right hand chakra, then place your right hand near the affected part. Maintain a distance of about three to four inches away from the patient. Continue concentrating or focusing your attention at the centers of your palms until the patient is sufficiently energized. For simple cases, this may take about five to fifteen minutes for beginners.

4) When energizing or projecting prana, you must will or form an initial intention directing the projected prana to go to the affected chakra and then to the affected part. It is a critical factor that the projected prana be directed to the affected part; this will produce a much faster rate of relief and healing. Just energizing the affected chakra without willing or directing the pranic energy to go to the affected part would result in a slower distribution of prana or vital energy from the treated chakra to the affected part; thereby producing a much slower rate of relief and healing.

5) The left and right armpits should be slightly opened to allow easier flow of prana from one hand chakra to the other hand chakra.

6) There should be an initial expectation or intention to draw in prana from one hand chakra to the affected part and to project prana from the other hand chakra. Once the initial intention or expectation has been formed, there is no need to further consciously expect or will to project. The initial expectation and concentration on the two hand chakras causes prana to be automatically drawn in through one of the hand chakras and projected out through the other hand chakra.

7) It is important to concentrate properly on both the left and right hand chakras. Success depends upon this. To concentrate more on the projecting hand chakra and not to give the receiving hand chakra sufficient concentration would tend to weaken and exhaust the healer.

8) If you feel slight pain or discomfort on your hand while energizing, flick your hand to throw away the absorbed diseased bioplasmic matter. When energizing, the hand should be flicked regularly to throw away the diseased bioplasmic matter.

9) Energizing should be continued until the treated part is sufficiently energized. The affected part has enough prana if you feel a *slight repulsion* coming from the treated area or if you feel a *gradual cessation* of the flow of prana from your palm to the treated area. The flow of prana may feel like a warm moving current or just plain subtle moving current. The feeling of slight repulsion or cessation of flow is due to the equalization of pranic energy levels between your hand and the treated area. For beginners, energizing with prana may take five to fifteen minutes for simple cases and about thirty minutes for more severe cases.

10) Cross-check whether the treated area is sufficiently energized by simply *rescanning* the inner aura of the treated part. If it is not, then energize further until the treated part has sufficient prana.

11) If the treated part is highly overenergized, apply distributive sweeping to prevent possible pranic congestion. This is done by sweeping the excess prana with your hand to the surrounding area. Cross-check the result by scanning. If the treated part is slightly overenergized by three inches, then just leave it as is.

12) Prana or ki may also be projected through the fingers or finger chakras rather than through the hand chakra. The prana coming out from the

finger chakras is more intense. If the projected prana is too intense, the patient may feel pain and a boring or penetrating sensation that is quite unnecessary. It would be better to master energizing through the hand chakras before trying to energize through the finger chakras.

In energizing with prana, visualization is helpful but not necessary. Just relax and calmly concentrate on the hand chakras. The result will automatically follow. The technique is simple, easy, and quite effective. Try it and judge for yourself.

In drawing in prana, there are several possible positions: Reaching for the Sky Pose, Egyptian Pose, and Casual Pose. In the Reaching for the Sky Pose, if you intend to draw in pranic energy through the left hand chakra, raise your left arm and turn the palm upward as shown in figure 11 on page 44. The act of raising the arm upward is like that of unbending a water hose. There is a meridian or bioplasmic channel in the armpit area which is connected to the left and right hand chakras. The unbending of this meridian allows prana to flow with minimum resistance. The act of concentrating on the left hand chakra is like turning on the water pump. By concentrating on the left hand, the left hand chakra is activated and draws in a lot of prana since there was an intention or expectation to draw in rather than to project prana.

In the Egyptian Pose, if you intend to draw in pranic energy through your right hand chakra, bend the right elbow until it is almost parallel to the ground. The arm is moved slightly away from your body to make a small opening in your armpit area. This has the effect of unbending the meridians in the armpit area. The palm is turned upward. This conditions the mind to receive prana. (See figure 12a on page 44.)

In the Casual Pose, if you intend to draw in pranic energy through your left hand chakra, let your left arm hang loosely and casually. The arm is moved slightly away from the body to allow a small opening in the armpit area. The palm is in casual position and is not raised upward. (See figure 12b.) The casual position requires more concentration for beginners since the upward position of the palm which conditions the mind to receive prana is not used.

I usually use the Egyptian Pose because it is more comfortable and does not look too strange. This reduces resistance from the patient. It is quite possible for a patient to partially and unintentionally block most of the prana projected to him by the healer if he finds the healer too strange or if he strongly rejects and disbelieves this form of healing. That is why it is better to establish rapport with the patient to make healing faster and easier.

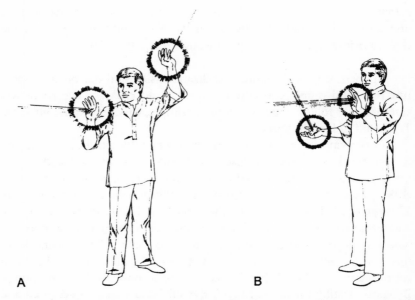

Figure 11. (A) Energizing with the Reaching for the Sky Pose; (B) energizing with the Egyptian Pose (standing position).

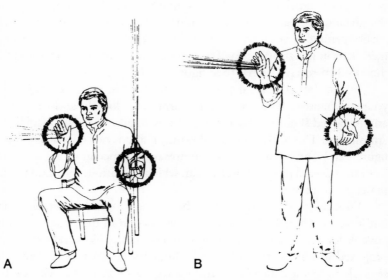

Figure 12. (A) Energizing with the Egyptian Pose (sitting position); (B) energizing with the Casual Pose.

STABILIZING THE PROJECTED PRANA

One of the potential problems in pranic healing is the instability of the projected prana. The projected prana tends to gradually leak out, causing possible regression or causing the illness to recur. This potential problem can be handled by thoroughly cleansing or sweeping the part to be treated and by stabilizing the projected prana. The projected prana can be stabilized in two ways:

• You should finish all energizing with prana by projecting blue prana. This is done by visualizing and projecting light-blue prana on the treated part.

• You can also just will or mentally instruct the projected prana to remain or stabilize.

You can perform this experiment to prove to yourself the validity of these principles and techniques. Use the following procedure:

1) Using the energizing-with-prana technique: project white prana on top of a table for about one minute and simultaneously visualize and form it into a ball without willing it to remain. This is the first pranic ball.

2) Project, visualize and form a blue pranic ball for about one minute without willing it to remain. This is the second pranic ball.

3) Project and form a white pranic ball for about one minute, and will or mentally instruct the pranic ball to remain for one hour. This is the third pranic ball. Make sure the locations of the pranic balls are properly marked and that there are no strong winds that might blow the balls away.

4) Scan the three pranic balls to make sure that they are properly formed.

5) Wait for about twenty minutes and scan the three pranic balls again. You may find that the first pranic ball is already gone or greatly reduced in size while the second and third pranic balls are still quite intact.

Please, do try this experiment immediately. It is simple and easy to perform.

BIOPLASMIC WASTE DISPOSAL UNIT

The diseased bioplasmic matter has to be disposed properly in order to maintain a bioplasmically clean room and to avoid contaminating yourself and the other patients from this dirty bioplasmic matter. The diseased bioplasmic matter, when removed from the patient's body, is still connected to the patient by bioplasmic threads. The Hawaiian shamans (healers) or *kahunas* call the bioplasmic thread invisible *aka* thread. In esoteric parlance, this is called etheric thread. Unless the diseased bioplasmic matter is properly disposed, there is the possibility that it may go back to the patient.

To make a bioplasmic waste disposal unit, simply get a bowl of water and add salt into the water. It has been clairvoyantly observed that water is capable of absorbing dirty bioplasmic matter and that salt breaks down the dirty bioplasmic matter.

After sweeping or cleansing, you should flick your hands toward the bioplasmic waste disposal unit. You can perform this simple experiment: get two bowls of water, put salt in one bowl and do not put salt in the other bowl. Scan the two bowls before and after flicking the dirty bioplasmic matter to each bowl. The dirty bioplasmic matter can be obtained from sweeping your patients. Leave the bowls for about two hours and note the difference. You will notice that you could hardly feel the diseased bioplasmic matter in the one with salt, but can still feel it in the one without salt.

Some healers use water, sand, water with tobacco, meat and other organic matters as bioplasmic waste disposal units. Some American Indian shamans use twigs. The twigs are placed in the mouth of the shaman and the diseased bioplasmic matter is sucked out or extracted by the use of the mouth. The twigs are used to catch the diseased bioplasmic matter.

The diseased bioplasmic matter is clairvoyantly and symbolically seen by some clairvoyants as spiders or insects or other repulsive forms. Some shamans do not place anything in their mouths. They just simply suck out the diseased bioplasmic matter and "dry vomit" it out. For beginners, there is the danger of literally swallowing the diseased bioplasmic matter. Therefore, it is safer to use sweeping.

PRACTICE TIME

The following schedule should be practiced for at least twelve days. This is to prepare you in case there is a sudden need to heal somebody, such as your own child. This practice should enable you to heal simple cases like fever, loose bowel movements, gas pain, muscle pain, insect and bug bites, etc.

Sensitizing the hands: five to ten minutes per day.
Scanning: five to ten minutes per day.
General and localized sweeping: ten minutes per day.
Energizing with prana: ten minutes per day.

Preferably, these techniques should be applied on actual patients. If this is not possible, then get a friend or relative to practice on.

If you are one of those few who are not able to sensitize your hands on the first session, just proceed to sweeping and energizing with prana. Continue the practice of sensitizing your hands. You should be able to accomplish it in three to four sessions.

It is advisable to learn to heal simple cases first before going to more difficult cases. This is necessary in order to gain experience and confidence. It is preferable to heal at least thirty simple cases before trying to heal difficult or severe cases.

THREE THINGS TO AVOID IN PRANIC HEALING

1) Do not energize the eyes directly. They are very delicate and are easily overdosed with prana if directly energized. This may damage the eyes in the long run. The eyes can be energized through the back of the head or through the area between the eyebrows. There is a chakra (energy center) in each of these locations. It is safer to energize through the ajna chakra (the area between the eyebrows). If the eyes are already sufficiently energized, the excess prana would just flow to other parts of the body.

2) Do not directly and intensely energize the heart for a long time. It is quite sensitive and delicate. Too much prana and too intense energizing may cause severe pranic congestion of the heart. The heart can be energized through the back of the spine near the heart area. In energizing the heart through the back, prana flows not only to the heart but to other parts of the body. This reduces the possibility of pranic congestion on the heart. If the heart is energized through the front, the flow of prana is localized around the heart area, thereby increasing the possibility of pranic congestion.

3) Do not apply too intense and too much prana on infants, very young children (2 years old and younger), or very weak and old patients. With infants and very young children, their chakras (energy centers) are still small and not quite strong. Very weak and very old patients have chakras that are also weak. Too much prana or too intense energizing has a choking effect on their chakras. This is similar to the choking reaction of a very thirsty person who drinks too much water in too short a time. The ability of very weak and old patients to assimilate prana is very slow. These types of patients should be energized gently and gradually. They should be allowed to rest and assimilate prana for about fifteen to twenty minutes before you attempt to energize them again.

If the solar plexus chakra (energy center) is suddenly overenergized, resulting in the choking effect on the chakra, the patient may suddenly become pale and may have difficulty breathing. *Should this happen, apply localized sweeping immediately on the solar plexus area. The patient will be relieved immediately.* This type of case is rare and is presented only to show the reader what to do in case something like this happens.

STEPS IN HEALING

1) Observe and interview the patient.

2) Scan the spine, the vital organs, the major chakras, and the affected parts.

3) Apply general sweeping.

4) Do localized sweeping in the affected areas.

5) Rescan the affected parts. In case of pranic congestion, scan to determine whether the congestion has been significantly reduced. For pranic depletion, scan to determine whether the inner aura of the affected part has become a little bigger or has partially normalized.

6) For simple cases, sweeping or cleansing is sometimes sufficient to heal the patient.

7) Energize the affected parts with prana.

8) Get feedback from your patient. If there is some pain left, ask for the exact spots and rescan those areas. Do more sweeping and energizing.

9) If the part is highly overenergized, do distributive sweeping to prevent possible pranic congestion.

10) Rescan the treated area to determine whether the affected area has been sufficiently decongested or energized. Thoroughness is the key to dramatic healing or very fast healing.

11) In pranic congestion, cleansing is emphasized. In pranic depletion, energizing is emphasized.

12) Stabilize the projected prana.

For beginners, it is better to scan before questioning the patient. This is to improve your accuracy in scanning. Scanning, like decision-making or other human faculties, can be influenced by suggestion. In scanning the patient, you should watch out for this possible flaw and try to recheck your findings. Figure 13 on page 50 shows the basic organs in the body. You will need to learn these, as you will better understand the possible problems if you know where the various organs are located in the body.

For simple localized illnesses, general sweeping may be skipped. For infectious diseases, general sweeping should be applied even if it is just a simple eye infection or cold because the whole body is more or less affected. In infectious diseases, the outer aura usually has holes. The rate of healing is much faster when general sweeping is applied on these cases than when it is not.

CAN YOU HEAL WITHOUT SCANNING?

If your ability to scan is quite limited, you still can heal without scanning. For simple cases, just ask the patient what part hurts or is causing discomfort. Then apply localized sweeping and energizing. For some severe type of ailments, there are patterns that can be followed. For instance, patients suffering from heart ailments usually have imbalanced or malfunctioning heart and solar plexus chakras. Therefore, cleansing and energizing these two chakras would greatly improve the condition of the patient. The heart should be energized through the back heart chakra.

Although you can heal without scanning, you would be much more accurate and effective if you use scanning. Sometimes some of the malfunctioning chakras are located far away from the painful or ailing part.

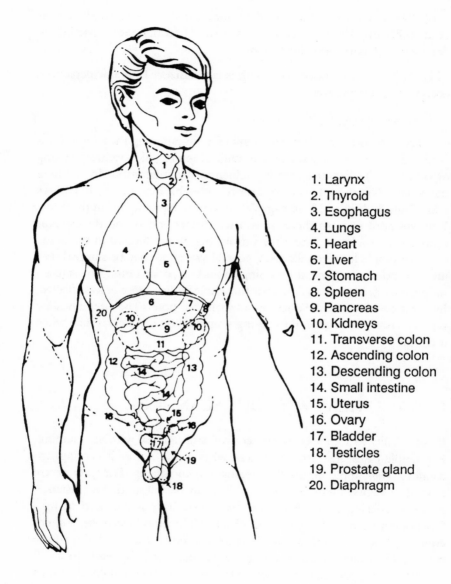

1. Larynx
2. Thyroid
3. Esophagus
4. Lungs
5. Heart
6. Liver
7. Stomach
8. Spleen
9. Pancreas
10. Kidneys
11. Transverse colon
12. Ascending colon
13. Descending colon
14. Small intestine
15. Uterus
16. Ovary
17. Bladder
18. Testicles
19. Prostate gland
20. Diaphragm

WASHING HANDS

Both hands, up to the elbows, should be thoroughly washed with water or salt water before healing, after sweeping, and after energizing. This washes away some of the diseased bioplasmic matter left on the hands of the healer and also reduces the possibility of absorbing it into your system. Otherwise, this may manifest as pain in your fingers, hands, arms or your patient's symptoms may manifest in your body. Washing is also necessary to prevent *bioplasmic contamination* on your next patient. Your hands should preferably be washed with germicidal soap to reduce the possibility of infecting yourself (the healer) or the next patient.

CRITICAL FACTORS IN HEALING

1) The patient must be scanned and rescanned thoroughly and accurately. Correct bioplasmic diagnosis will lead to correct treatment. Proper rescanning will give correct feedback as to the effectiveness of the initial treatment.

2) The patient's bioplasmic body must be thoroughly cleansed to increase the rate of healing and to avoid radical reaction.

3) The patient must be sufficiently energized with prana. Insufficient energizing means slight improvement or slow rate of healing. Overenergizing on delicate organs must be avoided to prevent pranic congestion.

4) Stabilize the projected prana to prevent it from escaping or leaking out. Many new healers become overconfident and commit the serious mistake of not stabilizing the projected prana when their patients tell them how their condition has greatly improved. As a result, some patients experience recurrence of symptoms or ailments after about thirty minutes or after a few hours. Therefore, always stabilize the projected prana after energizing!

5) Instruct your patients not to wash the parts that have just been treated for about twelve hours; otherwise, the symptoms may recur. Water absorbs some of the pranic energy that has been projected to the affected part. Patients suffering from severe ailments or general weakness are requested to refrain from taking a bath for about twenty-four hours after treatment.

This enables the body to gradually absorb and assimilate the pranic energy that has been projected.

CLOTHING

Materials such as silk, rubber and leather tend to act as partial insulators to prana. Patients should be requested not to wear silk since it makes it difficult to project prana on them. Leather or rubber shoes and leather belts should preferably be removed to make general sweeping more effective. Some healers also remove their shoes when healing in order to absorb more ground prana.

THE CHAKRAS

Although there are many major chakras, only seven of them will be discussed in this level. See figures 14 and 15 on the following pages for illustrations of the chakra locations.

1) *Basic or Root Chakra*: This chakra is located at the base of the spine or at the coccyx area. It energizes and strengthens the whole body and is responsible for your physical well-being. It energizes and affects the nearby organs and it also controls the adrenal glands. People with a highly activated basic chakra tend to be robust and healthy, while those who have less active basic chakras tend to be fragile and weak.

2) *Sex Chakra*: This chakra is located at the pubic area. It controls and energizes the sexual organs and the bladder.

3) *Solar Plexus Chakra*: There are two solar plexus chakras. The one located at the solar plexus is called the front solar plexus chakra and the one at the back is called the back solar plexus chakra. The term "solar plexus chakra" shall mean both the front and the back solar plexus chakras. The solar plexus chakra energizes and controls the pancreas, liver, stomach, large intestine, the appendix, the diaphragm and to a certain degree, the small intestine. The heart is greatly affected by this chakra. The front solar plexus chakra is an energy clearing house center, a large portion of prana from the lower chakras passes through the front solar plexus chakra before

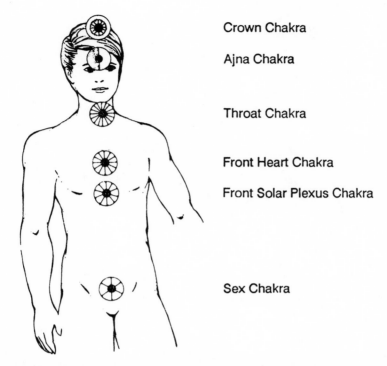

Crown Chakra

Ajna Chakra

Throat Chakra

Front Heart Chakra

Front Solar Plexus Chakra

Sex Chakra

Figure 14. The major chakras (energy centers) on the front of the body.

reaching the higher chakras and vice versa. The whole body can be strengthened by energizing the solar plexus chakra.

4) *Heart Chakra*: There are two heart chakras. The one located in front of the physical heart at the center of the chest is called the front heart chakra and the other is at the back and is called the back heart chakra. The front heart chakra controls and energizes the physical heart and the thymus gland. The back heart chakra controls and energizes primarily the lungs and to a lesser degree the heart and the thymus gland. The term "heart chakra" shall mean both the front and the back heart chakras.

5) *Throat Chakra*: The throat chakra energizes and controls the thyroid and parathyroid glands, and the throat.

6) *Ajna Chakra*: This chakra is located at the area between the eyebrows. It energizes and controls the pituitary gland, and it also energizes to a certain degree the brain. It is also called the *master chakra* because it directs

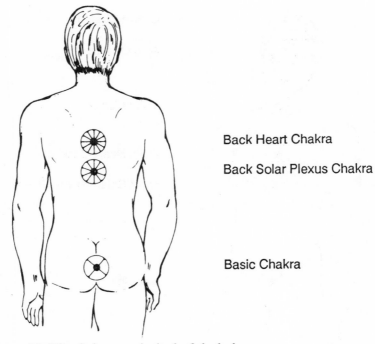

Back Heart Chakra

Back Solar Plexus Chakra

Basic Chakra

Figure 15. The chakras on the back of the body.

and controls the other chakras and their corresponding endocrine glands. Energizing this chakra will cause the other chakras to light in a certain sequence. Some healers project prana to the ajna chakra to reach an ailing part that is located far from the ajna chakra. The ajna chakra affects the eyes, nose, brain, and other nearby organs.

7) *Crown Chakra*: This chakra is located at the crown of the head. It energizes and controls the brain and the pineal gland. Energizing this chakra will cause the projected prana to flow to other parts of the body. It is just like pouring water to a funnel. Some healers project prana to the crown chakra in order to reach an affected part.

It is interesting to note that each of the seven major chakras energizes and controls an endocrine gland or glands.

The whole body can be energized through the crown, ajna, back heart, solar plexus, navel, spleen, basic, hand, and foot chakras. An affected part can be energized directly or through the nearest chakra. Some healers may energize through a farther chakra, such as the ajna or the crown chakra, to treat a heart or abdominal problem. Therefore, one can deduce that there are many possible healing techniques to treat one type of ailment. But the basic principles are the same—cleansing and energizing.

Acupuncture points and chakras are gates through which prana can easily go in or come out. By energizing through the nearest chakra, the projected prana will have easy and direct access to the affected part. Whereas, when energizing directly the affected part instead of through a chakra or chakras, a filtering action on the projected prana takes place; hence, energizing in this way takes more time and more prana.

In energizing the whole body, the solar plexus chakra is usually used because of its proximity to the many important organs in the body. It is located at the center of the trunk which contains many essential organs. Energizing the solar plexus chakra should be done slowly and gently. Too much and too intense energizing could cause difficulty in breathing.

4

Treatments for Simple Cases

I HAVE TAUGHT MANY ordinary people how to heal, and they have become relatively proficient in just a few weeks time. Pranic healing is easy. It just needs an open mind and a little perseverance. The following treatments for simple cases will get you started practicing the techniques you have learned thus far.

HEADACHE

Scan the crown chakra, the ajna chakra, the back of the head, the entire head and neck. Headaches could be caused by pranic depletion or congestion on these parts. The eyes, the temples, and the solar plexus should also be scanned.

Apply localized sweeping and energizing on the crown chakra, ajna chakra, the back of the head, and on the affected head area. If the cause is due to pranic congestion, localized sweeping is usually sufficient to remove the pain. Or just ask the patient what is aching, and apply localized sweeping and energizing on the affected part.

If the headache is due to eye strain, then the ajna chakra, the eyes, and the temples should be cleansed and energized. The eyes are energized through the ajna chakra. If it is due to an emotional problem or stress, then the front solar plexus chakra should be cleansed and energized.

Remember to always get feedback from the patient and to always rescan the treated area to determine whether treatment has been done properly.

EYESTRAIN OR TIRED EYES

Scan the eyes, ajna chakra, and the temples. These are usually depleted. Apply localized sweeping on these areas. Rescan to determine whether the inner aura of the treated areas has increased in size. If the size has increased, it means cleansing has been successful.

Energize the eyes by energizing the ajna chakra with the intention that fresh prana will flow to the eyes. You must remember that energy or prana follows thought or where your attention is focused. Energize the temple areas.

TOOTHACHE

Scan the affected part. There is usually pranic depletion on the painful area. Clean the affected area by applying localized sweeping. Energize the affected part. Instruct the patient to see a dentist as soon as possible.

COLD WITH COUGH AND STUFFY NOSE

Scan the ajna chakra, the throat chakra, the front solar plexus chakra, the back heart chakra, and the lungs (front, sides, and back). These areas may be congested and/or depleted. See figure 16 for the chakras involved.

Since the whole body has been affected to a certain degree, apply general sweeping to clean the whole body. Then apply localized sweeping and energizing on the ajna chakra, throat chakra, back heart chakra, and

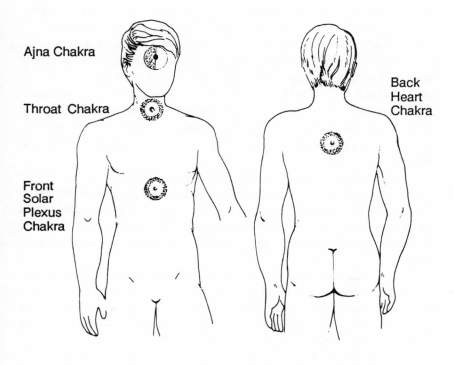

Ajna Chakra

Throat Chakra

Front
Solar
Plexus
Chakra

Back
Heart
Chakra

Figure 16. Pranic treatment for colds.

lungs. This is to clean and energize the respiratory system from the lungs
to the throat and up to the nose.

Apply localized sweeping and energizing on the front solar plexus
chakra. This is to energize and strengthen the whole body.

Rescan the treated areas and get feedback from the patient. If the
treatment has been done properly, the patient should be greatly relieved.
The patient may be given another treatment after four hours to reinforce
the earlier treatment and to ensure rapid healing.

Instruct the patient to rest and not to eat too much. Eating too
much consumes a lot of prana which is needed for the rapid healing of
the body.

FEVER

Scan the whole body with emphasis on the seven major chakras, the spine, the lungs, the abdomen, and the soles of the feet. People suffering from fever usually have small inner auras of about two inches or less.

Clean the whole body thoroughly by applying general sweeping four or five times. Clean and energize the hand chakras, and the sole chakras at the feet. (See figure 17.) This is to partially activate and energize the hand and sole chakras; thereby increasing their capacity to absorb ground and air prana. This will gradually and steadily energize the whole body, providing sufficient prana or vital energy to fight the infection.

Clean and energize the front solar plexus chakra and the navel. This is very important and is a critical factor in rapidly bringing down the fever. (See figure 18 on page 61 for chakra locations.) Fever is usually caused by pulmonary infection. If the throat chakra, the back heart chakra, and the lungs are affected, then apply localized sweeping and energizing on them.

When this technique is done properly, most patients will show dramatic improvement in an hour or less. On rare cases, some patients may experience a slight increase in temperature in the first two hours. This is partly due to the radical reaction and the intensified fight between the germs and the white corpuscles.

The treatment should be given two to three times a day to greatly increase the rate of healing. The patient is likely to recover in less than a day or two.

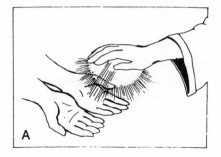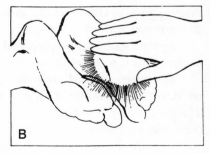

Figure 17. Pranic treatment for fever. (A) shows how to energize the hand chakras; (B) shows how to energize the feet.

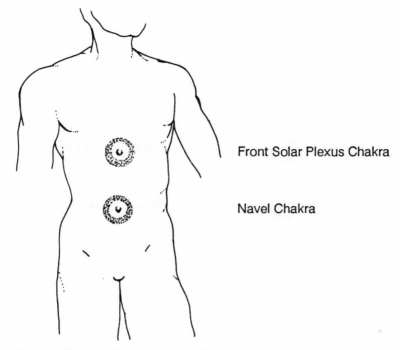

Front Solar Plexus Chakra

Navel Chakra

Figure 18. The chakras involved when treating fever.

STOMACH PAIN AND GAS PAIN

Scan the front solar plexus chakra, the navel and the abdominal area. Apply localized sweeping on the front solar plexus chakra, the navel and the abdominal area. Energize the front solar plexus chakra and the navel. If the pain is due to pranic congestion, most likely the patient will be partially if not fully relieved just by sweeping. (See figure 19 on page 62.)

DIARRHEA

Scan the front solar plexus chakra, the navel and the abdominal area. Apply general sweeping. Apply localized sweeping on the front solar plexus chakra, the navel and the abdominal area. Energize the front solar plexus

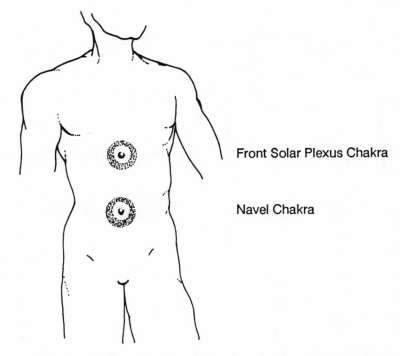

Front Solar Plexus Chakra

Navel Chakra

Figure 19. Pranic treatment for stomach pain, gas pain, diarrhea and constipation.

chakra and the navel. The patient should experience relief after a short duration of time.

CONSTIPATION

Scan the front solar plexus chakra, the navel, the abdominal area and the basic chakra. Apply localized sweeping and energizing with an emphasis on the front solar plexus chakra and the navel. (See figure 19.)

Usually the patient would be relieved in less than thirty minutes. For acute constipation and chronic constipation, it may take several hours before the patient will be relieved. This treatment, when applied regularly, will improve and strengthen the eliminative system.

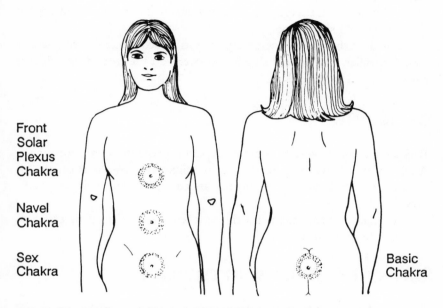

Figure 20. Pranic treatment for dysmenorrhea (menstrual cramps).

DYSMENORRHEA

Scan the sex chakra, the navel, the lower abdominal area and the basic chakra. Apply localized sweeping and energizing on the sex chakra, the navel, and the basic chakra. (See figure 20.)

If the patient is exhausted, then the front solar plexus should also be treated. Most patients will be relieved in a short time.

IRREGULAR MENSTRUATION OR NO MENSTRUATION

Use the treatment for dysmenorrhea. Check the ajna chakra and the throat chakra.

MUSCLE PAIN AND SPRAIN

Apply localized sweeping and energizing on the affected part. The emphasis should be on energizing. Most patients will recover partially, if not completely, in a short time.

For a fresh sprain, energizing should be continued until there is complete relief. The patient should not overexert the treated part since it has not healed completely.

BACKACHE

Backache usually manifests as pranic depletion. Scan the spine thoroughly. Apply localized sweeping on the entire spine with emphasis on the affected part. Apply energizing on the affected part. The relief is usually very fast.

Repeat these treatments for the next few weeks. This is necessary to make the healing permanent.

DIFFICULTY IN RAISING THE ARM

This may be caused by pranic depletion or congestion in the armpit and the surrounding areas. Difficulty in raising the arm could also be caused by heart ailment or high blood pressure.

Scan the areas thoroughly. Apply localized sweeping and energizing on the armpit and on the shoulder. By thoroughly cleansing and energizing the armpit, most patients will experience dramatic improvement in just a few minutes. (See figure 21.)

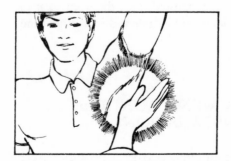

Figure 21. Pranic treatment for difficulty in raising the arm.

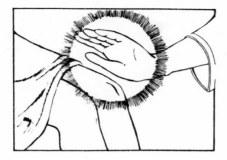

Figure 22. Pranic treatment for cuts, burns and concussions.

CUTS, BURNS, AND CONCUSSIONS

Apply localized sweeping immediately and energize thoroughly. Make sure the treated area is sufficiently energized. (See figure 22 for an example.)

Since the rate of pranic consumption is very fast, the treatment has to be repeated once every hour for the next three hours. Repeat the treatment twice a day for the next few days.

If the cut or concussion is on the head area, localized sweeping should be applied before and after energizing to avoid pranic congestion in the head area, which may cause headache or other unpredictable side effects.

When the treatment is done properly and thoroughly, the rate of healing is very fast and quite dramatic.

INSOMNIA

If the patient is too excited or overenergized, apply downward general sweeping four to seven times. This would be sufficient to make the patient drowsy. Apply downward sweeping only. Do not apply upward sweeping since it would tend to make the patient more alert.

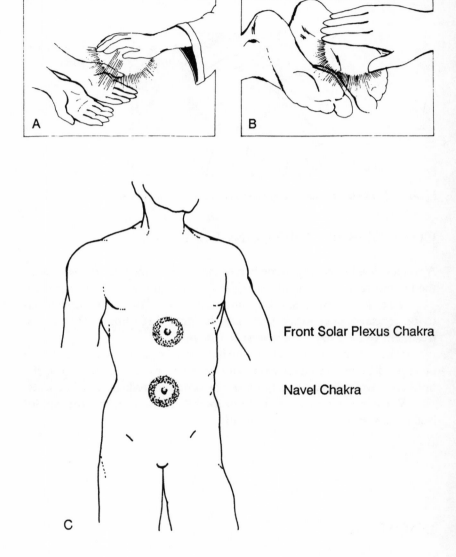

Front Solar Plexus Chakra

Navel Chakra

Figure 23. Pranic treatment for general weakness. (A) shows energy being sent to hand chakras; (B) shows energy to the feet; and (C) shows the body chakras that need energizing.

If the patient feels depleted, apply general sweeping about two times. Clean and energize the front solar plexus chakra. If the crown chakra is affected, clean and energize it.

GENERAL WEAKNESS

Apply general sweeping two times. (See figure 23 on page 66.) Clean and energize the hand and sole chakras. This will partially activate and energize the hand chakras and the sole chakras making them absorb more ground and air prana, which will gradually and steadily energize the whole body. Rescan the hand and sole chakras to determine whether they have greatly increased in size.

Clean and energize the front solar plexus chakra and then the navel. Continue energizing until the patient feels much better.

INSECT AND BUG BITES

Apply localized sweeping. Energize intensely and sufficiently the affected area. There should be some reduction in redness and swelling in less than thirty minutes. Repeat the treatment after one hour.

BOILS

Apply localized sweeping and energizing on the affected part.

PIMPLES

Apply localized sweeping and energizing on the face. The face is depleted and the inner aura relatively grey. Scan the ajna and solar plexus chakra. Apply localized sweeping and energizing on these chakras. It seems pimples may have something to do with emotions and the pituitary gland.

The face may be treated once or twice a day while the major chakras may be treated once every two or three days. The patient is expected to watch his or her diet and to keep the face regularly clean. Irritating the pimple should be avoided.

The emphasis should be on cleansing and energizing the face. Substantial improvement may occur in a few weeks time.

HICCUP

Clean and energize the front solar plexus chakra. Energizing should be continued until the patient is relieved.

NOSEBLEED

Clean and energize the ajna chakra and the root of the nose. Continue energizing until the bleeding stops.

STIFF NECK

Scan the lower back part of the head, the entire neck, the shoulder, and the armpit. Apply localized sweeping and energizing on the affected lower back part of the head, the affected part of the neck, the nape, the affected shoulder, and the affected armpit. If the right area is painful, then the right lower back part of the head, the center and the right part of the neck, the nape, the right shoulder, and the right armpit should be cleansed and energized thoroughly.

The emphasis should be on the lower back part of the head, the neck and the nape. If done properly, the effect is quite dramatic. Stiff neck could also be caused by heart ailment or high blood pressure.

MUSCLE CRAMPS

Scan the affected part. Apply localized sweeping thoroughly. Apply energizing on the affected part. The emphasis should be on energizing. Energizing should be continued until there is substantial or complete relief.

FREQUENCY OF HEALING

Many of you will wonder how often you should work on a patient. There are several things that you must think about. First of all, you must consider the severeness and the criticalness of the ailment. In severe cases, the rate of deterioration could be quite fast. For healing to take place, the rate of healing must be faster than the rate of deterioration. To increase the rate of healing, the frequency of the treatments has to be increased. For example, in treating patients with cancer, the treatment has to be given at least once a day or once every two days. If the treatment is given once every two weeks, the patient is not likely to improve because the rate of deterioration is much faster than the rate of healing.

In emergency or critical cases, the rate of deterioration is so fast that the treatment may have to be given once every hour or once every four hours depending upon how urgent the case is. In acute appendicitis, the treatment has to be given once every hour for the next four hours or until the condition has substantially improved. The treatment should be given two to three times in the next few days. Not all cases of acute appendicitis can be healed by pranic healing. Some may require surgery.

The next thing you need to consider is the rate of pranic consumption. Tissue damages, such as burns, cuts, concussions, and acute infections consume a large quantity of prana at a very fast rate. If the patient is suffering from severe infection or burn, then the affected part should be energized once every hour for the next few hours since the rate of pranic consumption is very fast. In acute pancreatitis, the patient can be treated once every four hours until you see substantial improvement. Another factor to consider is how fast the patient wants to get well. If a patient has a bruise on the arm and wants to get well in a day or two, this would require several applications of pranic healing for the first few hours. If healing is done immediately and properly, the skin will not blacken or turn yellow and the rate of healing would be very fast, less than a day or two at most.

If the patient just wants a moderate rate of healing, then the treatment can be applied just once. If pranic healing is applied immediately, then the concussion will be healed within a few days.

You must also consider *the delicateness and importance of the part being treated*. If the organ being treated is quite delicate and vital, such as the head, eyes, or heart, then healing should preferably be applied at longer intervals to avoid any possible pranic congestion for it could have serious consequences. If the part being treated is not so delicate or sensitive, such as the knee or the arm, then healing can be applied once every hour for the next four hours without serious side effects or radical reactions.

The age and health condition of the patient is another thing to consider. Patients who are very weak, old or very young require a series of mild treatments since their ability to absorb prana is very slow.

These are just some of the factors to be considered in determining the frequency of treatments. The healer should use sound judgment or discrimination on this matter. I prefer to treat a patient at an interval of once every two to three days in most cases. In critical cases or if the patient wants a very fast rate of healing, pranic treatment is applied once every hour for the next few hours on the first day and once or twice a day for the next few days. It is necessary to observe or monitor the patient closely for possible radical reactions for they could be serious.

HOLISTIC APPROACH IN HEALING

As I have said earlier, disease can be caused by internal or external factors or a combination of both. Obviously, the health condition of a person is dependent upon the well-being of the visible physical body, the bioplasmic body, and the psychological health of the patient. Although many of the simple and serious diseases can be healed by pranic healing, it is better to reinforce the healing process by taking herbs or medicinal drugs. If the visible physical body and bioplasmic body are treated simultaneously, obviously the rate of healing would be much faster and more effective than orthodox medicine alone or pranic healing alone. An acupuncturist uses acupuncture to treat the bioplasmic body and herbs to heal the visible body by strengthening the affected organs. Although I only use pranic healing and have obtained amazing results, I do not discourage or prohibit my patients from taking medicine or undergoing surgery. The ancient famous Chinese doctor Hua To was noted not only for his skills in acupuncture and herbs but also for his surgical skills.

Although pranic healing can do a lot of fantastic things, it has its limitations. Sometimes proper diet, physical exercise, taking herbs or medicinal drugs, a change in lifestyle, emotional therapy or surgery is required. It is important to maintain one's objectivity and have a proper perspective of what the different types of healing can do. Extremes and fanaticism should be avoided. Just as it is foolish for doctors trained in orthodox medicine to ignore or sometimes ridicule paranormal healing, it is equally foolish for a pranic healer to ignore what modern medicine is capable of doing and what it has done to cure and alleviate suffering.

HOW DO YOU WILL?

You do not have to tense your muscles or exert extraordinary effort when you "will" or exert your intent. You do not even have to visualize or close your eyes. When you perform with understanding, expectation, and concentration, you are already willing! The degree of concentration required is not extraordinary. The degree of concentration used in reading a book is sufficient to perform pranic healing. I do not expect you to believe or disbelieve what I have written. What is expected from you is an open, inquiring mind with a strong interest to experiment with and verify the validity of the principles and techniques suggested in this book.

LEVEL TWO:
INTERMEDIATE
PRANIC HEALING

Man lives only as long as he has vital energy in his body. If he lacks vital energy, he dies. Therefore, we should practice pranayama [controlling vital energy through breathing].

—Hatha Yoga Pradipika

By rhythmic breathing and controlled thought you are enabled to absorb a considerable amount of prana, and are also able to pass it into the body of another person, stimulating weakened parts and organs and imparting health and driving out diseased conditions.

—Yogi Ramacharaka
The Science of Psychic Healing

5

Drawing in Prana

WHEN YOU BEGAN THIS STUDY, you learned to draw in prana through one of the hand chakras. Now you will learn pranic breathing in order to absorb or draw in tremendous amounts of prana through the whole body from your surroundings. There are many types of yogic breathing that are used for different purposes. Yogic breathing that enables the practitioner to draw in a lot of prana and facilitates the projection of prana is called pranic breathing.

PRANIC BREATHING

When you do pranic breathing, it energizes you to such an extent that your auras temporarily expand by 100 percent or more. The inner aura expands to about eight inches or more, the health aura to about four feet or more, and the outer aura to about six feet or more. All of these can be verified through scanning. (See figure 24 on page 76.)

Why not try this simple experiment: ask a friend to do pranic breathing for about five minutes. Scan your friend before he starts, and after he

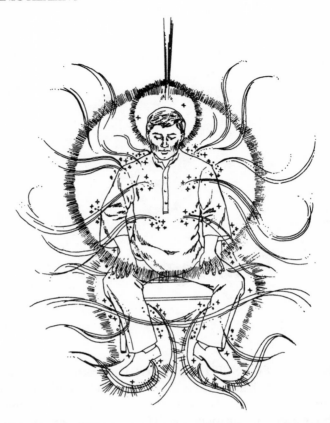

Figure 24. Pranic breathing. By doing pranic breathing you are able to absorb and project tremendous amounts of vital energy or prana.

has done pranic breathing for about two minutes. Note the changes in the sizes of the auras. You may even feel a rhythmic pulsation or expansion. It is important that you perform this and other experiments so that your knowledge will be based on solid foundations.

Method 1: Deep Breathing with Empty Retention

1) Do abdominal breathing.

2) Inhale slowly and retain for one count.

3) Exhale slowly. Retain your breath for one count before inhaling. This is called empty retention.

Method 2: 7-1-7-1

1) Do abdominal breathing.

2) Inhale for seven counts and retain for one count.

3) Exhale for seven counts and retain for one count.

Method 3: 6-3-6-3

1) Do abdominal breathing.

2) Inhale for six counts and retain for three counts.

3) Exhale for six counts and retain for three counts.

Abdominal breathing expands your abdomen slightly when inhaling and contracts your abdomen slightly when exhaling. Do not over-expand or over-contract your abdomen. This would make breathing unnecessarily difficult. (See figure 25.)

The critical factors are the rhythm and the empty retention. Holding your breath after exhalation is called *empty retention*; and holding your

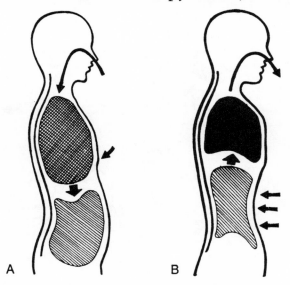

Figure 25. Abdominal breathing: (A) inhaling; (B) exhaling.

breath after inhalation is called *full retention*. Through clairvoyant observation, it is noted that there is a tremendous amount of prana rushing into all parts of the body when inhalation is done after empty retention. This does not take place if the inhalation is not preceded by empty retention.

When drawing in prana, you may use either pranic breathing or the hand chakra technique or both simultaneously.

DRAWING IN GROUND, AIR AND TREE PRANA

There is a minor chakra in each foot. This chakra is called the sole chakra. By concentrating on the sole chakras and simultaneously doing pranic

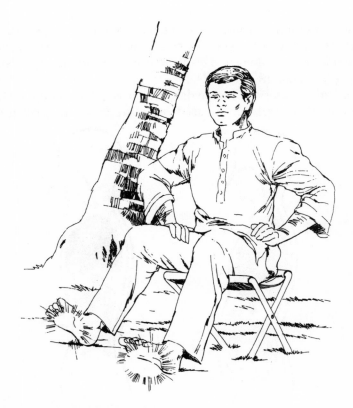

Figure 26. Drawing in ground prana.

breathing, you can tremendously increase the amount of ground prana absorbed through the sole chakras. (See figure 26.) Concentrating on the sole chakras activates them to a certain degree. Pranic breathing greatly facilitates or helps the sole chakras in drawing in ground prana. Drawing in ground prana is one way of energizing yourself. Ground prana seems to be more effective in healing the visible physical body than air prana. For example, wounds and fractured bones seem to heal faster with ground prana than air prana.

This technique of drawing in ground prana or earth ki is practiced in Chinese esoteric martial art, known as ki kung, the art of generating internal power.

1) Remove your shoes. Leather shoes and rubber shoes reduce the drawing in of prana by 30-50 percent.

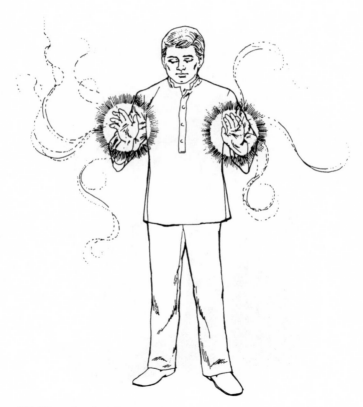

Figure 27. Drawing in air prana.

2) Press the hollow portion of your feet with your thumbs to make concentration easier.

3) Concentrate on the soles of the feet and do pranic breathing simultaneously. Do this for about ten cycles.

You can use the same principle to draw in air prana or tree prana through the hand chakras to energize yourself. To draw in air prana through the hands, just concentrate on the hand chakras and simultaneously do pranic breathing. (See figure 27.) To draw in tree prana through the hand chakras, choose a big healthy tree and ask mentally or verbally the permission of the tree to draw in its excess prana. (See figure 28.) Put your hands on the trunk of the tree or near it. Concentrate on the center of your palms and simultaneously do pranic breathing. Do this for ten

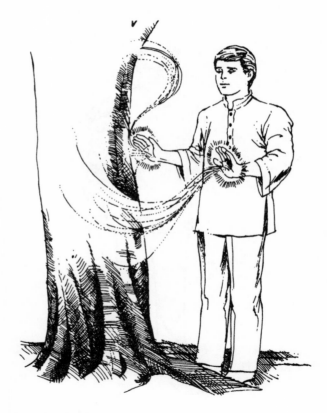

Figure 28. Drawing in tree prana.

cycles and thank the tree for the prana. Some of you may experience numbness or a tingling sensation throughout the body. Once esoteric principles and techniques are fully explained, they are usually very simple.

After energizing yourself, it is advisable to circulate the prana throughout the body. Visualize yourself filled with light or prana and circulate the prana continuously from the back to the front several times, then from the front to the back several times also.

SENSITIZING THE HANDS THROUGH PRANIC BREATHING

By now, most of you should have more or less permanently sensitized your hands. However, sometimes you may experience moments when the hands seem unable to feel or scan. This can be immediately remedied by concentrating simultaneously on the center of your palms and on the tips of your fingers while doing pranic breathing for about three cycles. This will cause the hand chakras and finger chakras to be activated, energized and sensitized so that you can scan accurately with your palms and with your fingers.

SCANNING WITH THE FINGERS

After sensitizing your hands, scan your own palm with your two fingers. Move your fingers slowly and slightly back and forth to feel the inner aura of your palm. Try to feel the thickness of your palm with two of your fingers and try to feel the different layers of the inner aura. Also practice scanning your palm with one finger. Always concentrate on the tips of your fingers when scanning with your fingers. This will activate or further activate the mini finger chakras; thereby sensitizing the fingers.

When scanning with your palms and fingers, always concentrate at the center of your palms and at the tip of your fingers. This will cause the hand and finger chakras to remain activated or to become more activated, thereby making the palms and the fingers more sensitive.

Being able to scan with the palms is not sufficient. You must learn to scan with your fingers. This is required in locating or proper scanning of small trouble spots. It is difficult to scan properly for small trouble spots with the palm because it may only feel the healthier surrounding areas around the small troubled spot. The small trouble spots are sometimes camouflaged by the healthier parts.

For instance, a person with eye problems usually has pranic depletion in the eyes, while the inner aura of the surrounding areas may be normal. Since the palm is quite big and the inner aura of the eyes is about two inches in diameter, it is likely that the palms may feel only the healthy eyebrows and forehead without becoming aware of the small trouble spots. This could be avoided if the fingers were used in scanning. The spinal column should also be scanned by using one or two fingers in order to locate small trouble spots.

In scanning a patient, you do not have to scan the outer and health auras. You were taught how to scan these auras in order to prove to yourself the existence of these auras. What is important is scanning the inner aura of the patient. In scanning the inner aura, it is important to feel the general energy level or the general thickness of the inner aura of the patient. This general energy level will be used as a reference or standard for comparing the conditions of some of the major chakras and vital organs. The accuracy of scanning will be affected if that area is scanned for too long because the scanned area will become partially energized.

It is important that you should be able to feel the pressure when scanning in order to determine the thickness of the inner aura of the part being scanned. Some of you may feel pain in your hands or fingers when in contact with a diseased part. The inner aura has several layers. In scanning the inner aura, you may feel pressure at about five inches and denser or stronger pressure at another layer about two or three inches away from the skin. Sometimes the inner aura of a part may seem normal. But when scanned further within, the next layer will seem rather thin, which means that the part is depleted. In scanning the inner aura, it is important to scan not only its first layer but also its inner layers. An advanced yogi or an advanced practitioner of ki kung has an inner aura that is comparatively big and has many layers. Sometimes the inner aura is more than three feet in thickness.

Scanning is also very useful in determining whether an infant or a child has a hearing or eyesight problem.

In treating serious cases, the eleven major chakras, the relevant minor chakras, all the major and vital organs, and the spine should be scanned thoroughly. It is through proper scanning and correct understanding of the nature of the ailment that the correct treatment can be determined.

SWEEPING WITH PRANIC BREATHING

General and localized sweeping is more effective when used with pranic breathing since more bioplasmic matter and prana are harnessed to remove diseased bioplasmic matter. When doing pranic breathing, the healer becomes more powerful because the etheric body (or bioplasmic body) becomes brighter and denser.

Just follow the instructions given in the first level of study for applying general and localized sweeping, and simultaneously do pranic breathing. With this type of sweeping, the patient is cleansed and energized simultaneously to a substantial degree. This type of sweeping is quite effective and very often sufficient to heal simple ailments. Sweeping can be done several feet away from the patient and with fewer strokes. You do not have to bother what hand position to use.

You may visualize luminous white prana sweeping and washing the patient from the crown to the feet when doing downward sweeping. Visualize the health rays being straightened. You do not have to do upward sweeping unless the patient is quite sleepy or has weak legs. When doing the upward sweeping, you may visualize the ground prana going up from the sole chakras to the crown chakra. This should be done after the patient has been cleansed sufficiently with downward sweeping. Applying upward general sweeping before applying downward sweeping may result in transferring diseased bioplasmic matter to the head and brain areas. This may result in serious harm to the patient, so don't do it.

You may or may not visualize when you do sweeping. For some healers, sweeping is more effective when accompanied by visualization. What is important is the intention to clean and energize the patient's bioplasmic body.

In sweeping, special attention should be placed on the back bioplasmic channel or the governor meridian[3], which interpenetrates the spine, and the front bioplasmic channel or functional meridian, which is opposite to the spine. Except for the spleen chakra, almost all the major chakras are located along these two channels or nadis. Cleansing or applying localized sweeping on these two channels would clean the major chakras located along these two meridians resulting in a much faster rate of healing. You

---

[3]Students should obtain a good acupuncture chart or a book on the subject so that you can become familiar with the meridians. The functional meridian is also known as the Triple Warmer.

must remember that all the major and vital organs are energized and controlled by the major chakras.

When applying localized sweeping, visualize the fingers and the hands penetrating into the diseased part and the grayish diseased matter being removed.

ENERGIZING WITH PRANIC BREATHING

Prana is drawn in by using pranic breathing and projected through one or both of the hand chakras. You can practice the following exercise to energize yourself and others.

1) Do pranic breathing slowly for about three to five cycles and simultaneously calm and still your mind.

2) Continue doing pranic breathing and simultaneously put your hand or hands near the part to be treated. Concentrate on the center of your palm or palms.

3) Will or direct the projected pranic energy to the affected chakra, then to the affected part. This is a critical factor, and in many cases would produce rapid relief since the affected part or organ will be quickly provided with sufficient pranic energy. Your attention should be primarily focused on the hand chakra (or chakras) and on directing the pranic energy, and less on the breathing.

4) Stop energizing when you intuitively sense the patient has enough prana or vital energy. Rescan the patient to determine whether he or she is sufficiently energized. In level 1 (or elementary pranic healing), you were instructed to stop energizing when you feel a slight repulsion or a cessation of flow of energy. As you become more advanced in healing, this guideline is no longer valid because your pranic energy level becomes much higher compared to that of the patient. To equalize your pranic energy level with the affected part of the patient may result in pranic congestion on the part being treated.

5) If the patient has severe infection, burns, or cuts, then the treatment has to be repeated after half an hour or an hour. These cases consume

pranic energy at a very fast rate; therefore, the treatments have to be repeated more frequently.

6) For pranic healers who are in the process of becoming proficient, relieving simple ailments may require five to seven breathing cycles and more serious ailments may require about twelve cycles or more. This is just to give you a rough idea. You may energize using your palm chakras or your finger chakras or both simultaneously.

Energizing should always be done simultaneously with pranic breathing. It is preferable to do pranic breathing for three to five cycles before you start energizing and to continue pranic breathing for two cycles after you have stopped energizing. This is to prevent possible general pranic depletion on the part of the healer.

Double Energizing

There are two types of double energizing or energizing with two hands: parallel double energizing and non-parallel double energizing. See figures 29 and 30 (on page 86). In parallel double energizing, simply place your hands facing and parallel to each other with the affected part in between

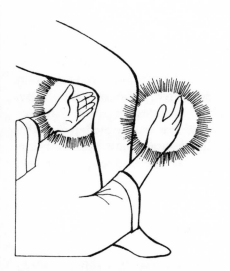
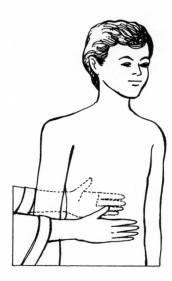

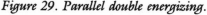
Figure 29. Parallel double energizing.

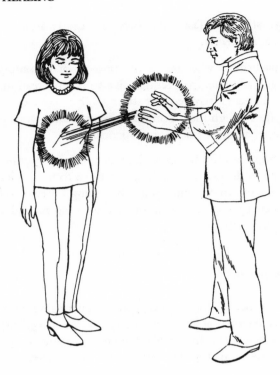

Figure 30. Non-parallel double energizing.

them. In non-parallel double energizing, your hands are directed at the affected part but are not parallel to each other. In parallel double energizing, an intense energy field is created causing the hand to rhythmically expand and contract. A tingling sensation is felt, not only in the affected part, but also in other parts of the body. At times the patient may even feel a slight electric shock. Double energizing is usually used in cases that require a tremendous amount of prana. Cleansing must be done before double energizing. Double energizing can also be used to quickly relieve simple ailments or illnesses mentioned in level 1.

Energizing: Distributive Sweeping Technique

Energizing with the use of the distributive sweeping technique simply means the use of sweeping to redistribute excess prana from other parts of the body to the ailing part:

1) Clean the ailing part by applying localized sweeping.

2) Sweep the excess prana with your hand from the surrounding parts and chakras to the treated part.

This type of energizing is quite effective in healing simple ailments. But is not so effective in more serious cases since these types of ailments require a tremendous amount of prana.

DISPOSING DISEASED BIOPLASMIC MATTER

There are times when it is inconvenient or not possible to throw the diseased bioplasmic matter into a bioplasmic waste disposal unit. Should this happen, just simply visualize a fire beside you and throw the diseased bioplasmic matter into the fire. Then extinguish the visualized fire after treating your patient. You can also will the diseased bioplasmic matter to disintegrate when you flick it away. These two techniques are to be used only by more advanced healers.

For beginners, you can try to heal in open spaces and throw the diseased bioplasmic matter into the ground. It is a common practice among shamans to dispose of objects filled with diseased bioplasmic matter by burning them, exposing them in the air for prolonged periods of time or burying them underground.

UTILIZING GROUND PRANA IN HEALING

There is a greater concentration of prana just above the ground than in the air. The density of prana just above the ground is about four or five times greater than the prana contained in the air. This concentration of ground prana can be used for healing.

Ask your patient to lie down on the ground. A cotton blanket or a mat made of natural material may be used to lie on. Avoid using leather, rubber, synthetic foam, a synthetic mat or blanket, for they tend to act as insulators, which hinder the free flow of ground prana into the body.

Apply general sweeping and localized sweeping several times. Let the patient rest and gradually absorb the ground prana. The act of cleansing causes a sort of partial "pranic vacuum" that results in the rushing of ground prana into the bioplasmic body of the patient and into the treated part. Energy tends to flow from greater intensity to lower intensity or from greater concentration to lower concentration. Once the patient is cleansed, energizing from ground prana occurs automatically and gradually. The healer should preferably energize the patient after sweeping to shorten the time required to substantially energize the affected part.

This is also the reason why some shaman healers go to the extent of burying the patient in the ground so that he or she can absorb more ground prana. If one is not feeling too well, one can take a swim in the sea for ten to fifteen minutes to cleanse the bioplasmic body and after that bury his or her body in the sand to gradually absorb ground prana.

RELEASING THE PRANIC ENERGY FOR HEALING

A healer will notice that it is easier to be detached when healing strangers than when healing one's own children, relatives, or close friends. This is caused by the healer's tendency to be too anxious about the results, due to the emotional attachment with the patient. Clairvoyantly, this attachment is seen as an etheric or energy cord linking the healer to the patient. Because of this cord, the projected prana may return to the healer; therefore, the patient may get well slowly, instead of rapidly.

It is important for the healer to be calm and detached, but at the same time thorough, when healing. After treatment, the healer should visualize the etheric cord as being cut. This disconnects the etheric link that causes projected pranic energy to bounce back to the healer.

Furthermore, if the patient is very depleted, there is a possibility that the healer will unknowingly continue to energize the patient even long after treatment. This will cause the healer to be depleted. Again, it is important to be detached when treating patients.

Healing will also be a lot easier if the patient is receptive to it—or doesn't offer strong resistance. Projected prana can be rejected by any patient if he or she is strongly biased against this type of healing, dislikes the healer, or does not really want to get well. It is advisable to establish a rapport with patients to reduce resistance. If there is strong resistance, request that the patient assume the receptive pose during the treatment. Ask the patient to turn his or her palms upward and bend the head slightly downward. Ask the patient to close his or her eyes. This reduces resistance and makes healing a lot easier.

To further increase receptivity, instruct the patient to mentally repeat several times during treatment the following affirmation: "I willingly, fully, and gratefully accept all the healing energy . . . in full faith, so be it!" You may also request that the patient mentally visualize his or her body and the affected part being filled with light (pranic energy).

PRACTICE SCHEDULE

Follow the schedule below for about two weeks. You should also try to treat many difficult cases. If you follow the instructions in this book consistently, your healing skill will develop very rapidly. You will be able to do a lot of things that may be considered by others as impossible or miraculous!

1) Scanning with two fingers—five minutes.

2) Pranic breathing and drawing in of air prana through the hand chakras—five minutes.

3) General sweeping at a distance of three feet from the patient—five minutes.

4) Energizing with pranic breathing—five minutes.

OTHER HEALING TECHNIQUES

The healing techniques that were explained earlier are those that I use. There are many other healing techniques used by other healers; however, the basic principles are the same—cleansing and energizing the affected parts. They are called extraction techniques (primitive, elementary, and advanced); short circuiting techniques (used for either cleansing and energizing or for the redistribution of prana).

Primitive Extraction Technique

There are several types of extraction techniques. The simplest form of extraction is done sometimes, if not usually, by natural born healers with no training in healing. These healers simply touch the affected part and involuntarily absorb or extract the pain and the diseased bioplasmic matter into the body without expelling it. They do not really know how to expel the diseased bioplasmic matter and do not understand what is happening. Consequently, they are affected by the diseased bioplasmic matter, but recover their energy after a good nights sleep. This technique is definitely not advisable.

Elementary Extraction Technique

Another type of extraction is accomplished by absorbing the diseased matter through one of the hand chakras and expelling it through the other hand chakra. You may use either of the hand chakras for extraction and expelling. Although this is an improvement over the primitive technique, it is still not advisable because there is always the possibility that some diseased bioplasmic matter will remain in the healer's body. Just imagine what would happen to the healer if he or she extracts dirty bioplasmic matter from twenty to fifty patients a day for two hundred fifty days a year. It is quite unlikely that the healer will remain healthy for long. He or she might even end up with many strange diseases. The idea of absorbing dirty, sticky, grayish diseased bioplasmic matter is just plainly repulsive.

Advanced Extraction Technique

Another type of extraction requires that the healer simply extract the diseased bioplasmic matter from the affected part by an act of will. The diseased bioplasmic matter is caught by the hand and flicked into the bioplasmic waste disposal unit. No sweeping movement is done. The hand is placed a few inches away from the afflicted part and the diseased bioplasmic matter is extracted by willing it to come out, but it is not absorbed.

Short Circuiting

Short circuiting can be done either to simultaneously clean and energize an afflicted part, or to redistribute prana from one area to another part. Short circuiting (cleansing and energizing) is done by simply placing the energizing hand at the back of the chakra to be treated and the extracting hand in front of it. This is done as follows:

1) Do pranic breathing.

2) Place your energizing hand at the back of the chakra to be treated.

3) Place your extracting hand in front of the chakra. Visualize your extracting hand surrounded by a layer of bright light.

4) Energize the back of the chakra. Visualize and will the dirty energy to come out. The diseased energy should not penetrate the layer of bright light on the extracting hand. Do not absorb the dirty energy into your body!

5) Flick the dirty energy into the bioplasmic waste disposal unit. The flicking of the dirty energy can be done at several intervals.

You can also use this technique to redistribute prana in the body. One hand is used for drawing in prana from the source and the other hand is used for energizing the part to be treated. For example, in treating an arthritic knee, the hand that is drawing in prana is placed in front of the basic chakra and the energizing hand is placed at the back of the arthritic knee.

ENERGIZING OBJECTS

Objects like water, food, herbs, medicine, alcohol, oil, ointment, balm, lotion, bandaids, bandages and cotton can be charged with prana to facilitate the healing process. Energized water can be taken internally by the patients—cold water absorbs more prana while warm water absorbs much less.

Herbs, drugs, ointments, balms, lotions and oil can be energized to increase their effectivity and potency. Rubbing alcohol can be energized to increase its disinfecting effect and to hasten the healing rate. Bandaids, bandages, and cotton can also be energized for similar purposes.

There are some patients who involuntarily or willfully resist the healing process. A patient that resists can, to a certain extent, block or prevent the entry of prana into the body. In this case, energized oil can be used as an entry point for prana. It acts as a gate or hole for prana to enter the patient's body.

For healing skin diseases, energized ointments, lotions or balms can be used after the initial pranic treatment. The number of healing sessions can be reduced because the healing process is compensated by the use of the energized ointment or medicine. Therefore the healer will have more time to treat more serious cases.

Objects can be energized by using pranic breathing and the energizing technique. Energizing can also be done by using physical means. It is quite likely that in a few decades from now, most drugs or medicines will be energized with prana to produce faster and more effective results.

6

Eleven Major Chakras

WE WILL NOW take a more advanced look at the chakras. Many students have been taught that there are only seven chakras, but in healing we shall work with lesser known chakras to create an extraordinary healing process. Figure 31 shows you the placement of the various chakras on the front of the body, while figure 32 shows the placement on the back of the body. As you experiment using these energy centers, you will find that they work quite well for you. For a breakdown of the chakras and how they relate to the various organs of the body and to disease, see Table 1 on pages 94–95.

The *crown chakra* is located on the crown of the head. It controls and energizes the pineal gland, the brain and the entire body. It is one of the major entry points of prana. Energizing the crown chakra has the effect of energizing the whole body. It is similar to pouring water in a funnel, causing the whole body to be flooded with prana. That is why some healers heal by energizing the crown chakra even though the affected part is somewhere else. Malfunctioning of the crown chakra may manifest as a disease related to the pineal gland and brain. These may also manifest as either physical or psychological illnesses.

The *forehead chakra* is located at the center of the forehead. It controls and energizes the pineal gland and the nervous system. Malfunctioning

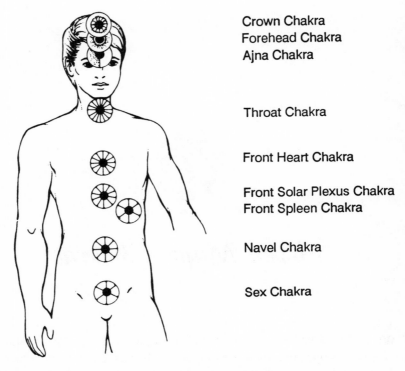

Crown Chakra
Forehead Chakra
Ajna Chakra

Throat Chakra

Front Heart Chakra

Front Solar Plexus Chakra
Front Spleen Chakra

Navel Chakra

Sex Chakra

Figure 31. The major chakras on the front of the body.

of the forehead chakra may manifest as loss of memory, paralysis and epilepsy. Energizing this chakra has a similar funneling effect like the crown chakra, causing the whole body to be flooded with prana.

The *ajna chakra* is located between the eyebrows. It controls and energizes the pituitary gland. It also controls or influences the endocrine glands and vital organs by controlling or influencing the major chakras. Malfunctioning of this chakra manifests as disease that relates to the endocrine glands and the eyes. Treating diabetes requires not only treating the solar plexus chakra (front and back), which controls the pancreas, but also the ajna chakra. Energizing this chakra causes the whole body to be energized. The mechanism is different from the crown and forehead chakra. Instead of the usual funneling effect, energizing the ajna chakra causes the other chakras to light up in a certain rapid sequence; thereby energizing the whole body. That is why in charismatic healing or invocative healing, the healers touch either the crown, forehead, or ajna chakra of

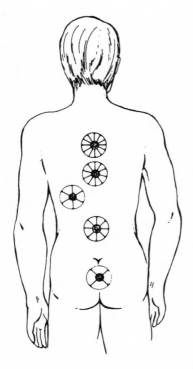

Back Heart Chakra

Back Solar Plexus Chakra

Back Spleen Chakra

Meng Mein Chakra

Basic Chakra

Figure 32. The major chakras and their placement on the back of the body.

the patient with their fingers or palms. The sudden intense rushing in of prana in the head area causes some patients to lose consciousness.

The *throat chakra* is located at the center of the throat. It controls and energizes the throat, the thyroid and parathyroid glands. To a certain degree it also influences the sex chakra. Malfunctioning of the throat chakra manifests as throat related illnesses such as goiter, sore throat, loss of voice, asthma, etc.

The *heart chakra* (front) is located at the center of the chest. It energizes and controls the heart, the thymus gland and the circulatory system. Malfunctioning of the front heart chakra manifests in heart and circulatory illnesses. The solar plexus chakra is quite sensitive to emotion, tension and stress, and has strong influence on the physical heart and the front heart chakra. Malfunctioning of the solar plexus chakra may cause the front heart chakra and the physical heart to also malfunction. The front heart chakra is closely connected to the front solar plexus chakra by several big bio-

Table 1. The chakras, the corresponding organs and possible diseases.

CHAKRA	LOCATION	FUNCTIONS AND CORRESPONDING ORGANS	DISEASES
1. Crown chakra	Crown of the head	Brain and pineal gland.	Diseases related to the pineal gland and the brain (physical or psychological illnesses).
2. Forehead chakra	Center of the forehead	Nervous system and pineal gland.	Loss of memory, paralysis and epilepsy.
3. Ajna chakra	Between the eyebrows	Pituitary gland and endocrine glands; controls the other major chakras.	Cancer, allergy, asthma, and diseases related to the endocrine glands.
4. Throat chakra	Center of the throat	Throat, thyroid and parathyroid glands.	Throat-related illnesses like goiter, sore throat, loss of voice, asthma, etc.
5. Heart chakra: a) Front heart	Center of the chest	Heart, thymus gland, and the circulatory system.	Heart and circulatory ailments.
b) Back heart	Back of the heart	Lungs, and to a certain degree the heart.	Lung ailments.
6. Solar plexus chakra:		Acts as an energy clearing house center. It also controls the heating and cooling system of the body.	
a) Front solar plexus	Solar plexus area or the hollow area between the ribs.	Pancreas, liver, diaphragm, large intestine, appendix, stomach, small intestine and to a certain degree other internal organs and other parts of the body.	High cholesterol, diabetes, ulcer, hepatitis, rheumatoid arthritis, heart ailments and other illnesses related to these organs.
b) Back solar plexus	Opposite the front solar plexus chakra	It has the same function as the front solar plexus chakra.	

Table 1 (cont)

CHAKRA	LOCATION	FUNCTIONS AND CORRESPONDING ORGANS	DISEASES
7. Spleen chakra		Spleen	
a) Front spleen	Left part of the abdomen between the front solar plexus chakra and the navel chakra. It is located at the middle part of the left bottom rib.	Major entry point for air prana or air vitality globule; energizes the other major chakras and the entire body.	Low vitality, weak body, and blood ailments.
b) Back spleen	Back of the front spleen chakra.	It has similar functions with the front spleen chakra.	
8. Navel chakra	Navel	Small and large intestines.	Constipation, difficulty in giving birth, appendicitis, low vitality and other diseases related to the intestines.
9. Meng mein chakra	Back of the navel	Kidneys, adrenal glands; energizes to a certain degree other internal organs; controls blood pressure	Kidney problems, low vitality, high blood pressure and back problems.
10. Sex chakra	Pubic area	Sexual organs, bladder and legs: it is the lower or physical creative center.	Sex-related problems and bladder ailments.
11. Basic chakra	Base of the spine	Adrenal glands and sex organs; it energizes the physical body—bones, muscles, blood, and internal organs; affects general vitality, body heat, and the growth of infants and children; center of self-survival or self-preservation.	Cancer, leukemia, low vitality, allergy, asthma, sexual ailments, back problems, blood ailments, growth problems and psychological disorders.

plasmic channels. It is also energized by the front solar plexus chakra to a certain degree. Patients with heart problems usually have malfunctioning solar plexus chakra.

There is also a *back heart chakra* which is located at the back of the heart. It primarily controls and energizes the lungs and to a lesser degree the heart and the thymus gland. Malfunctioning of the back heart chakra manifests as lung problems. Energizing of the heart is done through the back heart chakra. The whole body can also be energized through the back heart chakra.

Energizing the front heart chakra immediately energizes the physical heart. The main problem is that the vital energy or prana tends to localize or does not spread easily to other parts of the body, which may result in serious heart pranic congestion. That is why it is not advisable to intensely energize the front heart chakra for a prolonged period of time. Experienced pranic healers prefer to energize through the back heart chakra, which does not have localized effect on the physical heart. Excess prana can easily flow to the lungs and other parts of the body.

The *solar plexus chakra* (front) is located at the solar plexus area (or the hollow area between the ribs). It controls and energizes the pancreas, liver, diaphragm, large intestine, appendix, and stomach; and to a certain degree it energizes the small intestine, lungs, heart and other parts of the body. The solar plexus chakra is the energy clearing house center.

Subtle energies from the lower chakras and from the higher chakra pass through it. The whole body can be energized through the solar plexus chakra. On rare occasions, overenergizing this chakra may result in difficulty in breathing. Excess prana should be removed immediately. The solar plexus chakra also controls the heating and cooling system of the body. Malfunctioning of this chakra may manifest as diabetes, ulcers, hepatitis, heart ailments and other illnesses related to the organs mentioned. The *back solar plexus chakra* is located opposite the front solar plexus chakra. The back solar plexus chakra looks like and has the same function as the front solar plexus chakra. It is slightly smaller than the front solar plexus chakra.

The *spleen chakra* (front) is located on the left part of the abdomen between the front solar plexus chakra and the navel chakra. It is located at the middle part of the left bottom rib. It is the major entry point for air prana or air vitality globule; therefore it plays a vital part in one's general wellbeing. It energizes the other major chakras and the entire body by distributing the digested prana to them. The *back spleen chakra* is

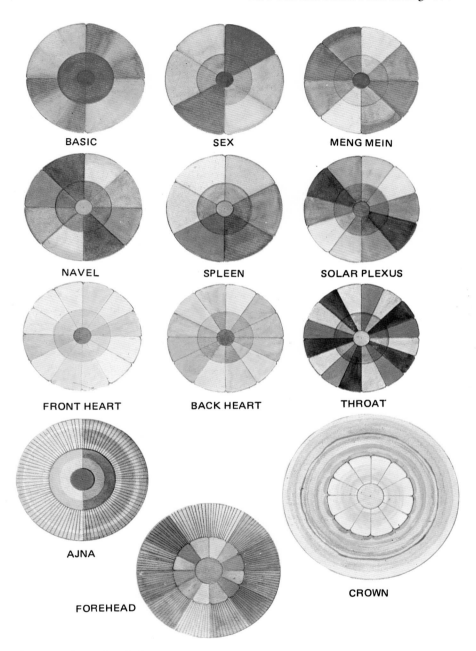

BASIC   SEX   MENG MEIN

NAVEL   SPLEEN   SOLAR PLEXUS

FRONT HEART   BACK HEART   THROAT

AJNA

FOREHEAD

CROWN

Plate 1. The major chakras.

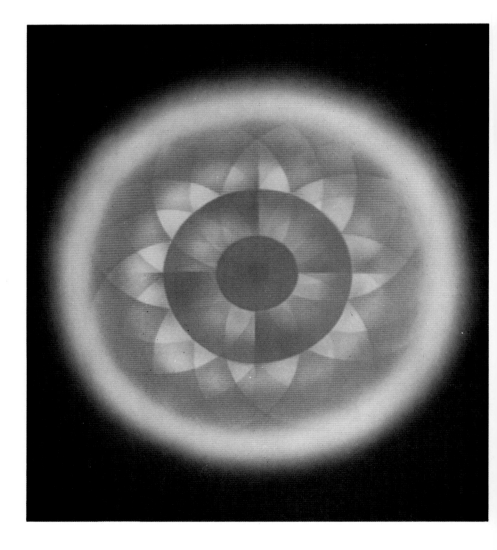

Plate 2. Basic chakra.

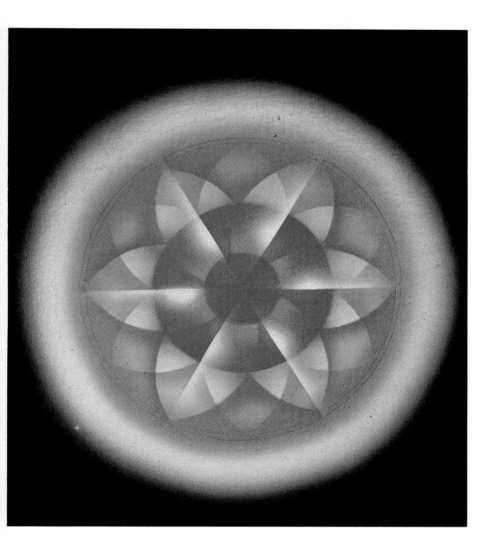

Plate 3. Sex chakra.

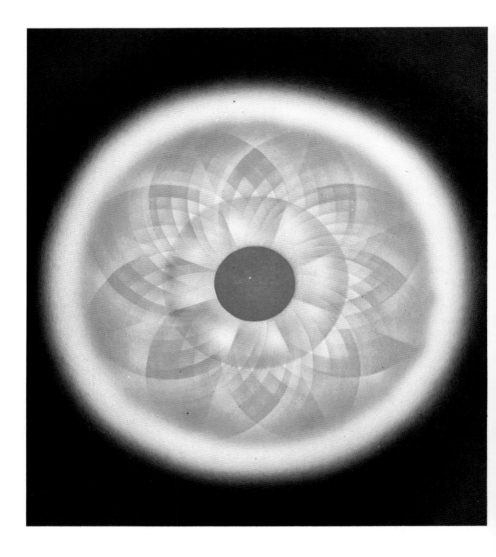

Plate 4. Navel chakra.

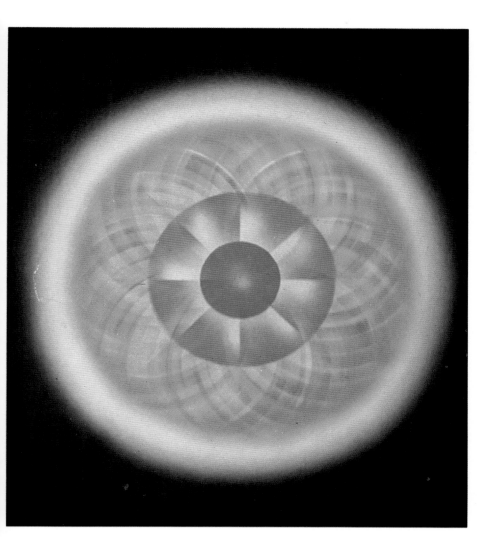

Plate 5. Meng mein chakra.

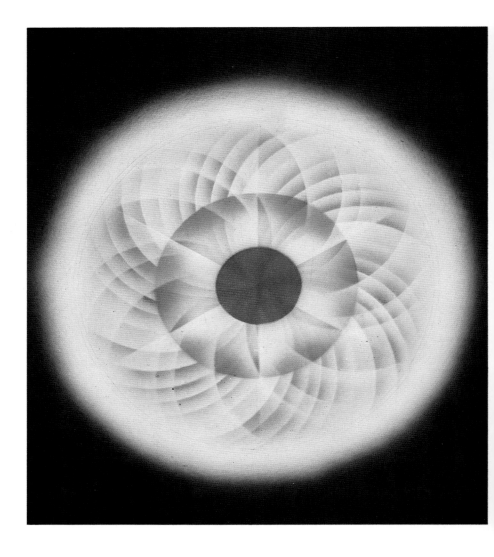

Plate 6. Spleen chakra.

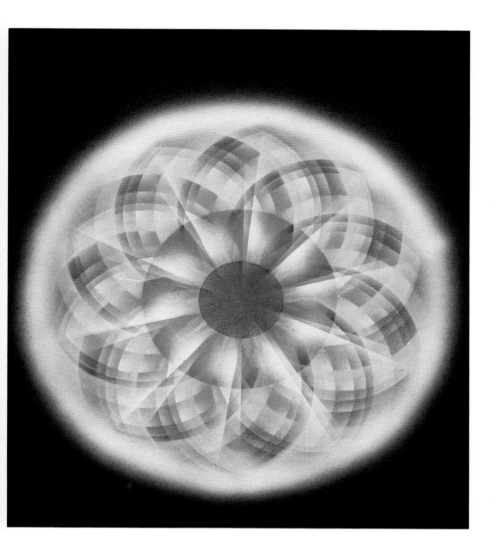

Plate 7. Solar plexus chakra.

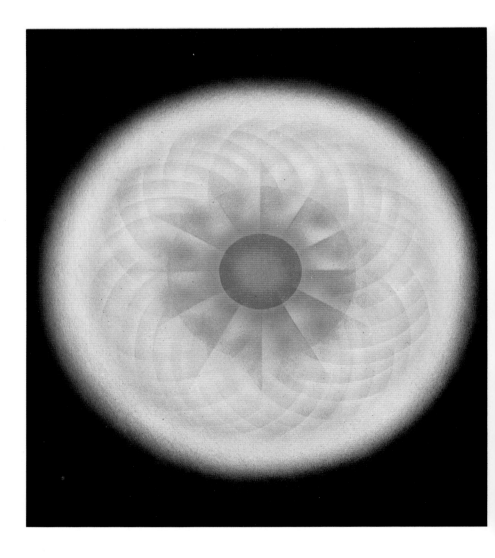

Plate 8. Front heart chakra.

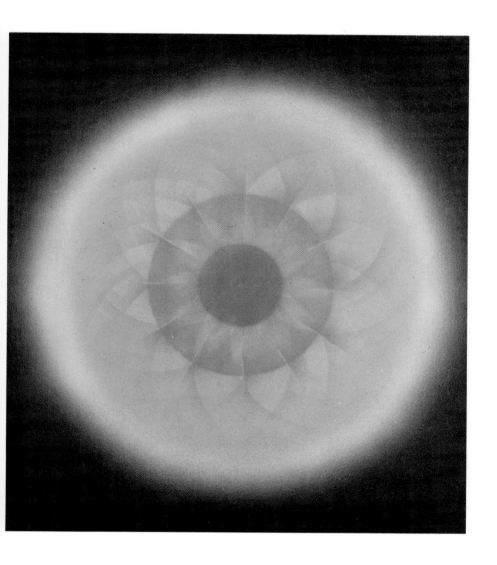

Plate 9. Back heart chakra.

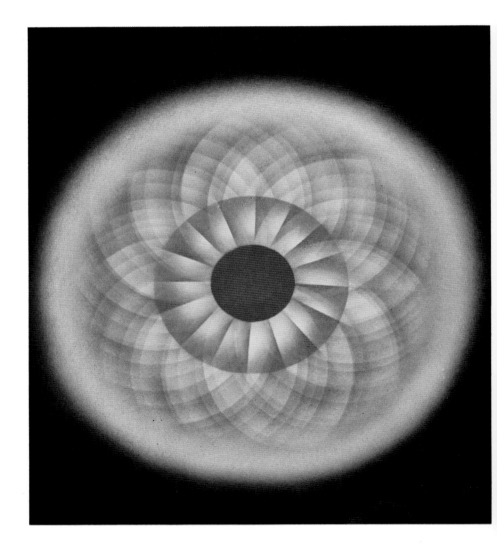

Plate 10. Throat chakra.

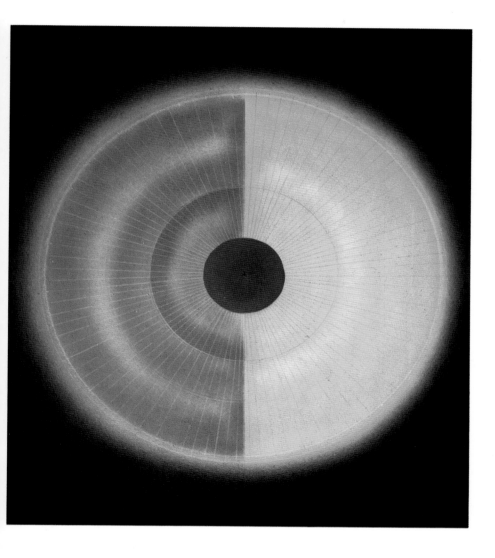

Plate 11. Ajna chakra.

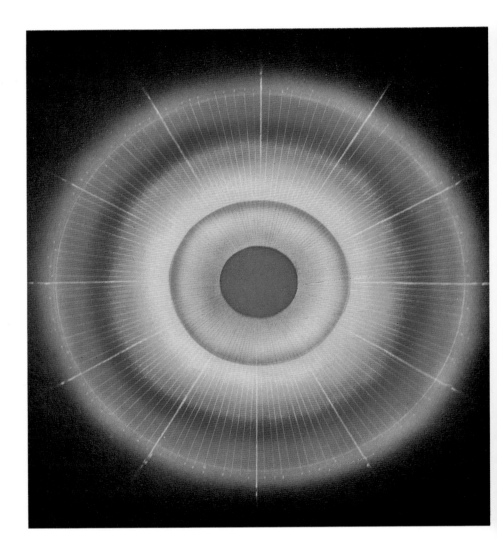

Plate 12. Forehead chakra.

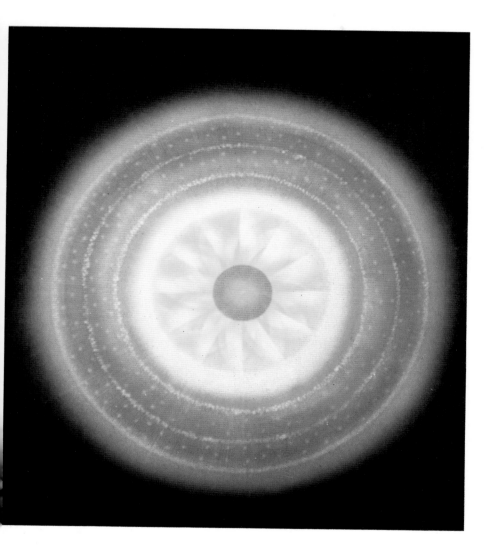

Plate 13. Crown chakra.

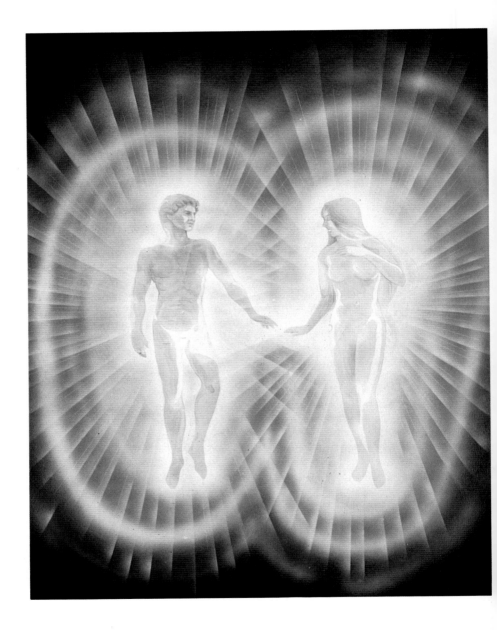

Plate 14 The inner and outer auras of a loving couple.

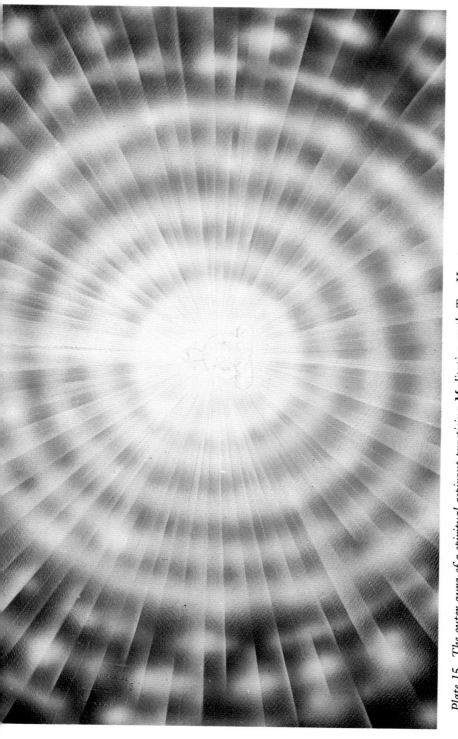

Plate 15. The outer aura of a spiritual aspirant practicing Meditation on the Two Hearts.

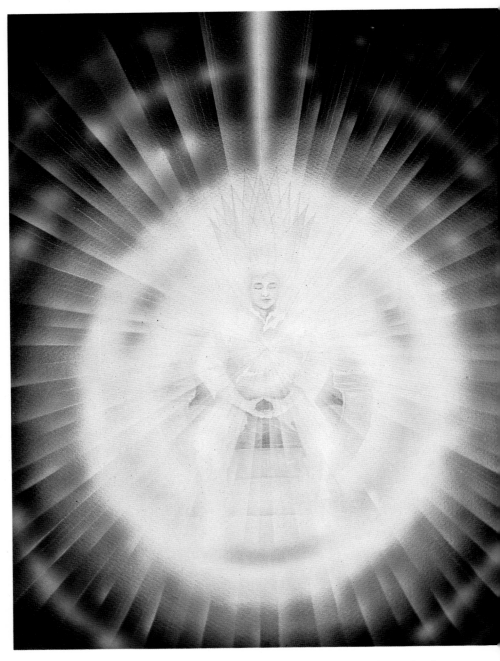

Plate 16. *Activated crown chakra of a spiritual aspirant practicing Meditation on the Two Hearts.*

located at the back of the front spleen chakra. The front and back spleen chakras have similar functions.

Please note: It is not advisable to energize the spleen chakra of infants and children because they may faint due to pranic congestion. Should this happen just apply general sweeping. It is also not advisable to energize the spleen chakra of patients with hypertension or a history of hypertension because this may increase blood pressure. However, this chakra is used to treat patients who are very weak or depleted. It is important that the spleen chakra should be treated by experienced or advanced pranic healers only.

The *navel chakra* is located on the navel. It controls and energizes the small intestine, lower large intestine, adrenal glands, and appendix. It affects the general vitality of a person. Malfunctioning of the navel chakra manifests as constipation, appendicitis, difficulty in giving birth, low vitality, and other diseases related to the intestines.

The word ki is used quite loosely to mean subtle energies. Ki is sometimes used to mean air prana, ground prana, red prana, and other types of prana. It is also used to mean a type of "synthetic ki" produced by the navel chakra. This "synthetic ki" is quite different from prana or vital energy. It affects one's ability to draw in, distribute, and assimilate prana. During bad weather conditions, the quantity of air prana is quite scarce. People with lesser "synthetic ki" have greater difficulty drawing in air prana; therefore they tend to feel rather tired or feel lower than the average person.

The *meng mein chakra* is located at the back of the navel. It serves as a "pumping station" in the spine that is responsible for the upward flow of subtle pranic energies coming from the basic chakra. It controls and energizes the kidneys, the adrenal glands and the blood pressure. Malfunctioning of this chakra manifests as kidney problems, low vitality, high blood pressure, and back problems.

The meng mein chakra of infants, children, pregnant women and older people should not be energized because of the serious adverse effects that will be produced. Please read about the master healing technique discussed elsewhere in this book for more explanation. This chakra should be treated only by experienced or advanced pranic healers.

The *sex chakra* is located in the pubic area. It controls and energizes the sexual organs and the bladder. Malfunctioning of this chakra manifests as sex related problems. The ajna chakra, throat chakra and basic chakra have strong influences on the sex chakra. Malfunctioning of any of these chakras may result in malfunctioning of the sex chakra.

The *basic chakra* is located on the base of the spine. It controls and energizes the whole visible physical body especially the bones, blood, muscles, tissues of the body and of the internal organs, adrenal glands, and sex organs. It affects body heat, general vitality, and the growth of infants and children. Malfunctioning of this chakra manifests as cancer, bone cancer, leukemia, arthritis, back problems, blood ailments, allergy, growth problems, and low vitality.

Treatments for Simple and Serious Cases

This chapter contains instructions for healing certain ailments. As I have said before, pranic healing can be used as a companion treatment when the patient is also seeing a medical doctor. You can also diagnose the aura and begin to treat for conditions that have not yet manifested in the physical body. The following treatments are not listed in alphabetical order; students should note that all treatments are listed in the index. Also, if you are not sure of the diagnosis, you can use the techniques described below in most cases.

WHAT TO DO WHEN YOU'RE NOT SURE

This technique is to be used by intermediate pranic healers. For simple or minor ailments:

1) Ask the patient about his complaint.

2) Apply sweeping and energizing twenty to thirty times on the affected areas.

3) Repeat treatment is necessary.

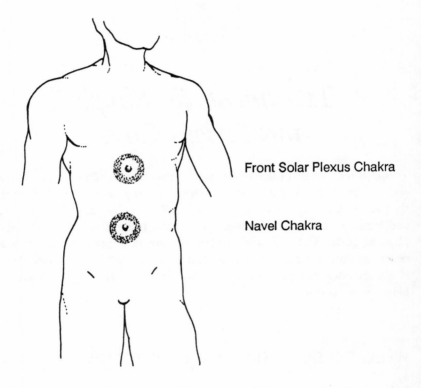

Front Solar Plexus Chakra

Navel Chakra

Figure 33. Increasing the body's defense system by increasing the vital energy level.

For more serious ailments:

1) Apply general sweeping several times.

2) Apply localized sweeping on all vital organs.

3) Apply localized sweeping and energizing on all major chakras except the spleen and the meng mein chakras. Do not energize these two chakras.

4) Repeat the treatment regularly.

You can use these procedures for many types of ailments, but instruct the patient to see a medical doctor immediately.

INCREASING VITAL ENERGY

Many ailments are due to bacterial and viral infections. By increasing the pranic or vital energy level of the body, its defense system is strengthened. (See figure 33.)

1) Apply general sweeping.

2) Clean and energize the sole and hand minor chakras. This is to partially activate the sole and hand chakras so they will absorb more prana, thereby increasing the vital energy level of the body.

3) Clean and energize the front solar plexus chakra. This energizes the whole body, especially the internal organs.

4) Clean and energize the navel chakra. This has two major effects: first, energizing and partially activating the navel chakra will cause the spleen chakra to be partially activated and energized so that it will absorb more prana, thereby increasing the vital energy level of the body. Second, the navel chakra is partially activated, thereby producing more "synthetic ki" which increases the ability of the etheric body to absorb more prana.

By increasing the vital energy of the body, the body's resistance or defense system is strengthened. This technique is used to rapidly bring down fever as taught in chapter 4.

MEASLES, GERMAN MEASLES, AND CHICKEN POX

1) Apply general sweeping.

2) Apply localized sweeping on the face, throat, and the front and back trunk. Special emphasis should be given to the abdominal area.

3) To increase the body's defense system, clean and energize the sole minor chakras, the hand chakras, the front solar plexus chakra, and the navel chakra.

4) Repeat the treatment once or twice a day. General sweeping and localized sweeping can be applied several times a day.

MUMPS AND TONSILLITIS

In order to work with these conditions, you will need to work with the throat and the jaw chakra. The jaw chakra is a minor chakra and is shown in figure 34.

1) Apply general sweeping.

2) Apply localized sweeping on the throat and entire neck area. Emphasis should be placed on the sides of the neck.

3) Energize the throat chakra.

4) Energize the jaw minor chakras which are located at the lowermost back part of the ears. By energizing the jaw minor chakras, the entire

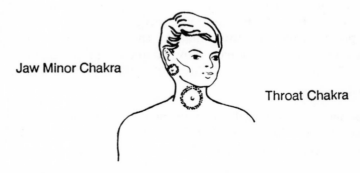

Figure 34. Pranic treatment for mumps and tonsillitis.

mouth will be energized including the parotid glands and the tonsils. Since the affected parts will consume prana at a very fast rate, the throat chakra and the jaw chakra should be cleansed and energized twice a day.

5) To increase the body's defense system, clean and energize the sole and hand minor chakras, the navel chakra, and the front solar plexus chakra.

FAINTING

1) Energize intensely the navel chakra until the patient recovers consciousness. This increases the pranic energy level of the whole body including the head area. This approach is slower but safer.

2) Another approach would be to energize the back of the head. This approach is faster but there is the possibility of pranic congestion of the head due to overenergizing. This manifests as headache.

3) If the loss of consciousness is due to sudden emotional shock, clean and energize the front solar plexus chakra and the navel chakra.

4) If head concussion is involved, clean and energize the affected part. Then energize the navel chakra, and the sole and hand minor chakras.

NEARSIGHTEDNESS, FARSIGHTEDNESS, AND ASTIGMATISM

There are minor chakras on each eye and on each temple. The ajna chakra, eye chakras and the temple chakras are usually depleted (pranic depletion). The thickness of these chakras usually ranges from two inches or less. In fewer or rare cases, you will encounter eye ailments caused by pranic congestion.

1) Scan the eyes, the ajna chakra and the temple chakras with one or two of your fingers. If the eye chakras are very depleted and have an inner aura of one inch or less, energize the eyes slightly through the ajna chakra by visualizing prana going to the ajna chakra then to the eyes before cleansing. This is to make localized cleansing or sweeping easier.

2) Apply localized sweeping or cleansing on the entire head, ajna chakra, eye chakras and temple chakras. If localized sweeping is done properly, the inner auras of the eye chakras would increase slightly.

3) Apply alternately energizing and localized sweeping on the ajna chakra, the eye chakras and the temple chakras until the inner auras of these chakras normalize in size and in density. The eyes should not be energized directly but should be energized through the ajna chakra. At times, you will feel that the inner aura of a treated part has increased to its normal size but is not sufficiently dense compared to other healthy parts. You should continue cleansing and energizing until the inner auras of the eyes, the temples and the ajna chakra are normalized.

4) It is quite likely that your patient will feel a slight immediate temporary improvement which is a good sign. The treatment should be repeated twice a week. Preferably, the patient should stop wearing eyeglasses to facilitate the healing process. Patients who suffer headache when they do not wear eyeglasses should gradually reduce the amount of time wearing them. Complete healing may take about three to four months.

CROSS-EYES AND WALLEYES

Apply the same treatment as the preceding case.

GLAUCOMA

The ajna chakra, eye chakras and the temple chakras are pranically depleted. If due to habitual stress or tension, the patient is likely to have a mal-functioning front heart chakra and solar plexus chakra.

During severe glaucomic attacks, the patient may experience intense pain in the head and eyes accompanied by general weakening. He or she may also experience blindness for a short or long period of time.

1) Scan the ajna chakra, eye chakras, temple chakras, heart chakras and solar plexus chakras.

2) To relieve the patient immediately of the pain or discomfort in the eyes, apply localized sweeping on the ajna chakra, the eye chakras and the

temple chakras. Energize the eyes through the ajna chakra until their conditions normalize. If done properly, the patient will experience a substantial degree of relief. For patients who are recently blind due to glaucoma, eyesight will be partially restored; for patients who have been blind for quite some time, restoring the eyesight may still be possible but will require longer treatment. The eyeballs may soften a little bit.

3) If the patient is experiencing a headache, scan the head area, and apply localized sweeping and energizing alternately to remove the headache.

4) If the patient is experiencing a general weakening of the body, apply general sweeping several times. Apply localized sweeping and energizing on the front solar plexus chakra. These will strengthen the patient and also make the relief last longer. The malfunctioning of the solar plexus chakra due to emotional stress is a major contributing factor to this ailment.

5) If the patient has a heart ailment, then the heart should also be treated.

6) Apply the treatment three times a week. This should be continued for several months or for as long as required. If the cause is of emotional origin, then hypnotherapy can be applied, or the patient can be taught how to relax and meditate in order to regulate emotions properly.

For a patient experiencing severe glaucomic attack, the treatment may be repeated after one or two hours if he or she is still experiencing discomfort. Instruct the patient to consult an eye specialist after the treatment.

HEART AILMENTS

Heart ailments may manifest as pranic depletion or congestion, or both simultanenously, in the heart chakra. Although there are many types of heart ailments, such as heart enlargement, malfunctioning of a pacemaker, partial failure of the heart muscles, etc., the treatment is basically the same and involves cleansing and energizing the heart chakra and the solar plexus chakra. See figure 35 on page 124.

1) Scan the heart thoroughly. Look for small trouble spots. Apply localized sweeping thoroughly on the front heart chakra and on the small trouble spots with your fingers. Visualize your fingers going inside the small trouble spots and removing the diseased bioplasmic matter.

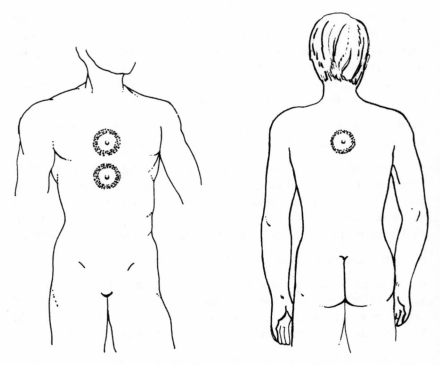

Figure 35. Pranic treatment for heart ailments. You will work with the front heart and solar plexus chakras, and the back heart chakra.

2) The heart should be energized through the back heart chakra and not through the front heart chakra. Visualize the physical heart and the front heart chakra becoming bright and clean. Get feedback from the patient to determine which spot or spots are still painful or uncomfortable. Rescan and apply localized sweeping and energize further. If done properly and thoroughly, the patient will experience immediate partial relief. Substantial relief may also be experienced after several hours or days. In pranic depletion of the heart, the emphasis should be on energizing, but thorough cleansing is also very important.

3) Apply localized sweeping and energizing on the front and back solar plexus chakras.

4) If there is severe pranic congestion in the front heart and front solar plexus chakras, then apply localized sweeping thoroughly. It may take five to ten minutes to thoroughly remove the congested diseased bioplasmic

matter. Usually, the patient will be relieved immediately after the localized sweeping. Energize the heart through the back heart chakra and apply more localized sweeping. Energize the solar plexus chakra and apply more localized sweeping.

5) If the patient is quite weak, general sweeping should be applied first before any other treatment in order to strengthen the health rays and to seal off holes in the outer aura. This will definitely make healing easier.

A treatment may last for a few minutes to about half an hour in most cases. Treatment should be applied three times a week. For critically ill patients, pranic treatment may be applied two or three times a day for the next few days. There are no fixed guidelines. You will have to use your own discretion.

It may take from several weeks to several months to heal and normalize the condition. The recovery period varies depending upon the seriousness of the heart ailment, the cooperation of the patient, the frequency of pranic treatment, and other relevant factors.

LUNG AILMENTS

There are many types of lung ailments (pneumonia, tuberculosis, etc.) but the treatment is more or less the same. (See figure 36 on page 126.)

1) Clean the entire body by applying general sweeping several times. Apply localized sweeping on the lungs (front, sides, and back) and on the back heart chakra. The lungs should be cleansed from all sides. If the front heart chakra is also affected, then it should also be cleansed.

2) Energize the back heart chakra and visualize prana going into all parts of the lungs. It is very important that the lungs and the back heart chakra be highly energized. If the heart is affected, visualize prana going into the heart and the front heart chakra. If the throat is affected, then it should also be treated. If the instructions are followed thoroughly, the patient will be relieved immediately and the tightness on the chest area will be greatly reduced.

3) Some patients with lung ailments are quite debilitated. To strengthen and increase the energy level of the body, clean and energize the front solar plexus chakra, navel chakra, plus the hand and sole minor chakras.

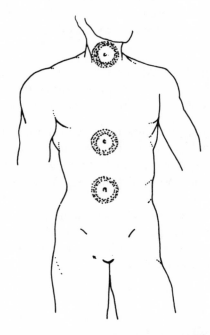

Figure 36. Pranic treatment for lung ailments. You will work with the throat, front solar plexus, and navel chakras as well as with the back heart chakra.

4) Apply pranic treatments twice a week until the patient fully recovers. For patients suffering from severe lung infection who are in critical condition, treatment should be given three times a day for the next few days.

ASTHMA

The treatment is divided into two parts. The first part is to relieve the patient from the asthmatic attack and to greatly improve and heal the respiratory system. The second part is to gradually remove the cause of the ailment. See figure 37.

1) The outer, health and inner auras of the patient are sometimes quite gray. It is advisable to apply general sweeping several times.

2) Patients suffering from asthma or asthmatic attack have a depleted throat chakra and secondary throat minor chakra. The secondary throat minor chakra is located on the lower soft portion of the throat. Apply localized sweeping and energizing on the throat chakra and on the secondary throat minor chakra. The emphasis is on energizing.

3) Clean and energize the back heart chakra and the lungs. This is to strengthen the lungs. If the solar plexus chakra is affected, clean and energize it. By treating the throat chakra, the back heart chakra and the solar plexus chakra, the patient will be immediately relieved.

4) An asthmatic patient has a malfunctioning ajna chakra and basic chakra. Clean and energize the ajna chakra and the basic chakra. To improve the quality of the blood produced, the bones in the body have to be cleansed

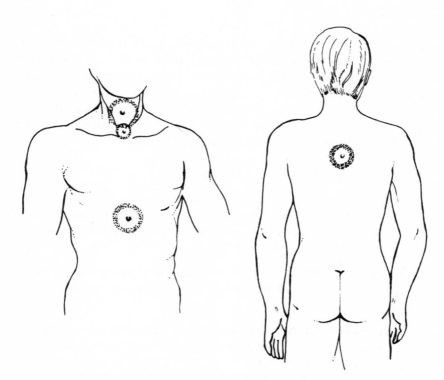

Figure 37. Treatment for asthma. You will use the throat chakra, the secondary throat chakra, the front solar plexus chakra and the back heart chakra.

and energized. Clean and energize the spinal column and the bones in the arms and in the legs. Apply localized sweeping and simultaneously energize the spinal column. Apply localized sweeping while visualizing your hand going into the bones of the arms and legs. Energize the bones in the arms through the armpit minor chakras and the hand chakras. Visualize pranic energy going into the shoulder blades and the bones in the arms. Energize the bones in the legs through the hip minor chakras and the sole chakras. Visualize the pranic energy going into the bones in the hips and in the legs. These will substantially reduce the frequency of the asthmatic attacks and will gradually cure the asthmatic patient.

5) Apply the entire treatment twice a week until the patient is cured.

LIVER AILMENTS

Patients with liver ailments such as jaundice, hepatitis or cirrhosis of the liver are quite depleted and have grayish inner, health, and outer auras. The liver, when seen clairvoyantly, is gray. If it is inflamed, then it is seen as muddy red. The liver may be depleted and congested simultaneously. For example, the left part may be congested while the right part is depleted. The solar plexus chakra is quite depleted (pranic depletion). Some patients with liver ailments have a bloated abdomen.

1) Apply general sweeping several times.

2) Apply localized sweeping and energizing on the solar plexus chakra and on the liver. In an area where there is pranic congestion, then localized sweeping should be emphasized. In an area where there is pranic depletion, energizing should be emphasized.

3) To increase the energy level of the body and to strengthen its defense system, clean and energize the sole and hand minor chakras, and the navel chakra.

4) If the meng mein chakra and kidneys are affected, clean and energize them. Do not energize the basic chakra because the patient may experience pranic congestion in the entire body or feel high blood pressure (see chapter 11 for further explanation).

5) Apply pranic treatment twice a week until healing is complete.

GASTRIC AND DUODENAL ULCERS

1) Scan the front solar plexus chakra and the upper abdominal area.

2) Clean and energize the front solar plexus chakra and the affected area.

3) Apply pranic treatment two or three times a week until healing is complete.

KIDNEY AND BLADDER INFECTIONS

1) Apply general sweeping several times.

2) If the kidneys are infected, clean the basic chakra, the meng mein chakra, and the kidneys. Then energize the kidneys directly without passing through the meng mein chakra.

3) If the bladder is affected, clean and energize the sex chakra.

4) Apply pranic treatment three times a week until healing is complete.

For infants, children, pregnant women, and older patients, do not energize the meng mein chakra. Just energize the kidneys directly without passing through the meng mein chakra. Overenergizing the meng mein chakra or energizing the basic and meng mein chakras may cause severe high blood pressure for this group of people. See figure 38 on page 130.

SEXUAL AILMENTS

1) There are many types of sexual ailments, such as impotence, infertility or prostate infections. To treat these types of cases, first scan the sex chakra, the navel chakra and the surrounding area. See figure 39 on page 130.

2) Clean and energize the sex chakra, the navel chakra and the affected surrounding area. There is a minor chakra in each of the ovaries and testes and if they are affected, clean and energize them.

3) Special attention should also be given to the basic chakra, the solar plexus chakra, the throat chakra and the ajna chakra. Malfunctioning of

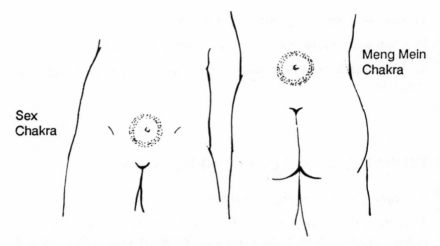

Figure 38. Treatment for kidney and bladder infections (read instructions thoroughly before applying).

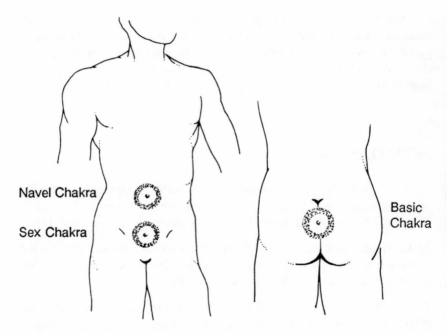

Figure 39. Treatment for sexual ailments.

any of these chakras will also cause the sex chakra to malfunction. If any of these chakras is malfunctioning, then localized sweeping and energizing should be applied.

4) Repeat the treatment twice a week until healing is complete.

AILMENTS OF THE ENDOCRINE GLANDS

1) Scan the major chakras.

2) Apply localized sweeping and energizing on the malfunctioning chakras. The ajna chakra should be treated.

3) Repeat the treatment twice a week until healing is complete. Instruct the patient to consult a specialist.

BROKEN BONES AND FINGERS

1) Scan the affected part and the affected minor chakras. There are minor chakras on the armpits, elbows, hands, fingers, hips, knees, soles and toes.

2) Apply localized sweeping and energizing on the injured area. Clean and energize the affected and/or the nearest minor chakras. The emphasis should be on energizing.

3) The nipple chakras affect the arms. They are located on each nipple. Scan the nipple chakra. If it is affected, then energize the nipple chakra. Prana can be easily directed to the affected area in the arm through the nipple chakra.

4) The healing process can be accelerated by increasing the pranic energy level of the body. Energize the basic chakra, the navel chakra, the solar plexus chakra, the hand chakras and the sole chakras.

You may repeat procedures 2 and 3 several times a day to quicken the healing process.

SMALL BREASTS

Women with small breasts may ask a pranic healer to activate and energize their busts if they are concerned about the size. Although the author has not personally tried this technique, he has observed that women with bigger breasts tend to have stronger or denser nipple chakras, while women with smaller busts tend to have weaker nipple chakras.

THINNING HAIR

A person may have a very healthy crown chakra and forehead chakra but still have thinning hair. This happens because the minor chakras on the scalp area are depleted. When scanning the head area, the initial layer of the inner aura on the head is quite normal but further scanning would show that the innermost layer is depleted. Clairvoyantly, this is seen as light gray or light yellowish gray in the scalp area. Apply localized sweeping and energizing on the entire scalp. Pranic treatment should be applied two or three times a week. Other complementary forms of treatments should also be given.

HEMORRHOIDS

Hemorrhoids manifest as pranic congestion on the anus minor chakra. The solar plexus chakra and the navel chakra are also partially affected. The anus minor chakra is located slightly above the anus and between the basic chakra and the anus. Clairvoyantly, it is seen as muddy red. Apply localized sweeping and energizing on the anus. The emphasis is on sweeping. Clean and energize the front solar plexus chakra and navel chakra. Visualize the prana cleansing and energizing of the large intestine. Visualize the prana coming out of the anus and cleansing the anus minor chakra. Treating the solar plexus chakra and the navel chakra is very important since the large intestine and the anus are controlled and energized by these two major chakras.

The patient may also use cold water to remove the diseased bioplasmic matter from the affected part. He just simply wills or intents that the cold water remove the diseased bioplasmic matter. The patient is also expected to maintain proper hygiene.

CHRONIC APPENDICITIS

1) Cleanse and energize the front solar plexus chakra, the navel chakra and the appendix. Usually, the patient will be relieved immediately.

2) Repeat the treatment once every two days.

SINUSITIS

1) Cleanse and energize the forehead chakra, the ajna chakra and the root of the nose. The emphasis should be on the ajna chakra.

2) Cleanse and energize the right and left nostril minor chakras. These minor chakras are located at the lower side of the nostrils.

3) Repeat the treatment twice a week.

LOSS OF SMELL

1) Use the treatment for sinusitis.

2) Check the ear chakra and the back head minor chakra. If they are affected, cleanse and energize them. It is likely that there will be noticeable improvement on the first treatment.

3) Repeat the treatment twice a week.

FREQUENT URINATION

1) Scan the patient thoroughly.

2) Apply localized sweeping and energizing on the sex, basic, navel, and solar plexus chakras.

3) Repeat the treatment twice a week for as long as necessary.

BED WETTING

For grown up children who are still bedwetting, apply the same treatment for frequent urination.

ENLARGED PROSTATE GLAND

Apply the same treatment for frequent urination. Repeat the treatment three times a week for as long as necessary. Instruct the patient to practice sexual abstinence during the duration of the treatment.

ARTHRITIS AND RHEUMATISM

For mild arthritis or rheumatism, just apply thorough sweeping and energizing to the affected parts. Repeat the treatment several times. In some cases, patients may feel relieved almost instantaneously. For severe cases of arthritis:

1) Apply general sweeping, then apply localized sweeping and energizing on the affected parts.

2) Apply localized sweeping on the liver, upper and lower abdominal areas.

3) Apply localized sweeping and energizing on the basic, navel, spleen, and solar plexus chakras. It is important that the basic chakra is energized thoroughly, since this chakra controls and energizes the skeletal and muscular systems of the body. Do not energize the spleen chakra if the patient is suffering from hypertension.

4) If the arm is affected, the entire arm has to be cleansed. The hand, elbow, and armpit minor chakras have to be energized. Do this to both arms.

5) If the leg is affected the entire leg should be cleansed and energized. Do this to both legs.

6) Repeat the treatment two to three times a week for as long as necessary.

PREGNANCY AND BIRTH

Pregnant women should be energized slowly and gently. Overenergizing or intense and prolonged energizing should be avoided—especially on the navel, sex, and basic chakras. Overenergizing or intense energizing on any of these three chakras may have drastic negative effects on the unborn child. The meng mein chakra should not be energized because if this chakra is intensely energized for a long time, the unborn child may be stillborn.

The treatment for pregnant women who have difficulty in giving birth is as follows:

1) Apply sweeping and energizing very gently on the navel chakra. This will ease labor and facilitate childbirth.

2) To reduce the pain, apply sweeping and energizing very gently on the sex chakra.

3) If her back is painful, apply sweeping on the lower back portion about four times. Do not energize the meng mein chakra.

To facilitate and hasten the recovery of a woman who has just given birth you would do the following:

1) Apply general sweeping.

2) Apply localized sweeping and energizing on the basic, sex, navel, and solar plexus chakras.

3) Repeat the treatment twice a day for five days. The mother should show remarkable improvement in two or three days.

There are ways to help prevent miscarriage. Women who have a tendency to miscarry have a depleted sex chakra and basic chakra. The navel chakra is partially depleted. The following treatment is applicable for women who are not pregnant but with a tendency to miscarry:

1) Apply general sweeping.

2) Apply localized sweeping and energizing on the sex, basic, navel, and solar plexus chakras.

3) Repeat the treatment twice a week for two months.

For pregnant women who have a history of miscarriage, and who are experiencing abdominal pain, the treatment is as follows:

1) Scan the body thoroughly.

2) Apply sweeping very gently on the navel, sex, and basic chakras, as well as on the abdominal area.

3) Energize the navel chakra and sex chakra very gently and slightly.

PRINCIPLE OF LAG TIME

The principle of lag time means that the rate of healing of the bioplasmic body is much faster than the rate of healing of the visible physical body. Therefore, in some cases the patient may not experience an immediate relief or cure because the visible physical body heals at a slower pace, or lags behind the bioplasmic body. For example, even though the heart area has been thoroughly cleansed, energized and looks quite bright, a patient may claim that he or she has experienced only very slight relief after the pranic treatment. However, substantial relief and improvement may be experienced after a few hours or after a day or two. This delay or lag time is especially common in more severe cases. The degree of delay or lag time will depend on whether there is organic damage or not, the degree of damage, the age and the condition of the patient's body.

HOW LONG TO COMPLETELY CURE A PATIENT?

This depends on several factors—the frequency of treatment, the age and physical condition of the patient, the patient's degree of receptivity, the presence of interfering or causal factors which delay or prevent healing from manifesting, the degree of damage, the nature of the ailment, the skill of the pranic healer, the degree of cooperation from the patient, and in some cases, the use of other forms of healing or treatment to complement pranic healing. As stated earlier, the approach in healing should be integrated or holistic.

The rate of relief for severe and simple ailments may range from a few minutes to a few days. In general, the time it takes to completely cure a simple ailment using pranic healing alone ranges from a few minutes to a few days; for chronic or more severe ailments, it may range from a few days to a few months. In some cases, the cure is even dramatic or miraculous. But not all ailments and not all patients can be cured.

IMMEDIATE RECURRENCE
OF PAIN OR SYMPTOMS

Several factors may contribute to the immediate recurrence of the symptoms after pranic treatment. For example, localized sweeping may not have been applied or energizing was not done sufficiently. When the part to be treated is not cleansed, fresh prana has difficulty penetrating fully into the part that is being treated. As I've said, it is like trying to put fresh water on a sponge filled with dirty water. This can be done by using a lot of prana and projecting it with a stronger force. However, there is the risk of radical reaction that will cause more temporary discomfort to the patient. It would be a lot easier if the dirty water is removed first from the sponge before pouring in fresh water.

Symptoms may recur if general sweeping is not applied on a patient with holes in the outer aura; therefore prana continues to leak out causing pranic depletion on the treated part again. Sometimes the projected prana is not stabilized, causing it to simply escape or leak out from the body.

If you do not use the bioplasmic waste disposal unit, the diseased bioplasmic matter is still connected to the patient's bioplasmic body. If the patient is not sufficiently energized, it may cause the diseased bioplasmic matter to be drawn back. And if the patient tries to recall or keeps recalling how his or her ailment feels, most likely the diseased bioplasmic matter may be attracted again to the bioplasmic body.

The patient may also suffer from a severe type of disease which consumes prana at a very fast rate and the prana projected by the healer was not sufficient. Therefore, the patient should be treated more frequently.

WHY SOME PATIENTS ARE NOT HEALED

All of the preceding factors mentioned (that may contribute to the immediate recurrence of pain or symptoms after pranic treatment) may also be contributing factors when patients do not get well. The patient may not be receiving the right pranic treatment due to improper scanning. For instance, difficulty in moving the arm could be caused by a pranic congestion in the heart chakra, the solar plexus chakra or the meng mein chakra. So just treating the arm will give temporary relief but not a permanent result.

Insufficient energizing and insufficient frequency of pranic treatment may be the reason the patient doesn't heal. This is like giving medication of insufficient dosage and at insufficient intervals.

Certain ailments may require other forms of treatment. For instance, ailments due to malnourishment or improper diet will require that eating habits be changed. Perhaps the patient is simply too old, too weak, or too sickly to be healed. For certain unexplained factors, some aged patients just do not retain a large portion of the projected prana. This does not mean, however, that old or sickly patients should be ignored. On the contrary, they should be given proper care and treatment.

You might also consider that the disease is of karmic origin and that the appropriate time for complete healing has not yet arrived. The patient may not have yet learned the lesson that he or she is supposed to learn. Books written on Edgar Cayce and his works provide a lot of information about karma in relation to disease.

PERSONAL HEALTH PROBLEMS YOU MAY ENCOUNTER

There are a number of health problems that you may experience. Some healers experience pain in the finger joints, or in the hands or arms. This is due to the absorption of diseased bioplasmic matter or disease etheric matter from patients. This can be avoided by immediately washing your hands and the arms after general and localized sweeping and also after energizing. In the long run, not washing your hands and arms immediately will result in a regular partial absorption of diseased bioplasmic matter that may result in arthritis of the fingers. You may use salt and water to wash your hands and arms.

Some healers may experience the symptoms or the ailments of their patients. This is due to full absorption of the diseased bioplasmic matter into your system. This could be caused by two factors: firstly, by not washing your hands and arms after healing; and, secondly, by not using the waste disposal unit when treating patients. Some of the diseased bioplasmic matter may have been absorbed through the legs from the surrounding area. It is advisable to take a shower after treating a lot of patients in one session to clean the entire body. The healer should wash the entire body with salt or with salty water. This process has a cleansing effect on the entire body and you will feel your body becoming lighter.

Some healers become sick with infectious diseases. This can be avoided by not healing when you are feeling low or after an emotional outburst or intense anger or irritation. These types of negative emotions cause temporary pranic depletion, drooping health rays and punctures on the outer aura. All these can cause the healer to be very susceptible to infectious diseases. It is also advisable to wash your hands and arms with germicidal soap. This is not only to protect the healer but also the next patient.

The healer may become too tired or depleted after treating a patient or several patients. This could happen because the healer energizes intensely and at a very fast rate. The amount of prana projected is much more than the amount of prana drawn in, or the rate of projecting prana is much faster than the rate of drawing in prana. This results in general pranic depletion. This can be avoided by being patient and by not being in a hurry. Heal your patients slowly and gradually.

Some healers have very high energy levels. The inner aura is about six feet or more in thickness and very dense. They can absorb a tremendous amount of prana at a very fast rate. But these are exceptional cases, not the general rule. Some healers are born with a very high energy level while others attain this through disciplined esoteric training. A certain type of lifestyle may also result in a very high energy level in the long run. By being a vegetarian most of the time, having a moderate sex life, living a well-regulated emotional life, possessing a clear prudent but decisive mind, and doing plenty of regular physical exercise (especially tai chi and yogic exercise) will result in good health and a very high energy level.

Through clairvoyant investigation, it is observed that vegetarians usually have a more refined bioplasmic body and a brighter and denser inner aura. Although it is advantageous to become a vegetarian, it is not a necessity.

After treating patients, some healers may continue "energizing" their patients subconsciously. This can be avoided by visualizing the cords between you and your patient as being cut off after the treatment. The healer is closely surrounded by his or her patients and they tend to draw in prana from the healer subconsciously, causing the healer to become depleted. This can be remedied by keeping a certain distance from the waiting patients. It is advisable for healers to take regular restful vacations to recharge his or her body.

RATE OF VIBRATION OF THE BIOPLASMIC BODY

The rate of vibration of the bioplasmic body of one person may differ from others. It may be higher or lower. If the bioplasmic body of the healer has a higher rate of vibration than that of the patient, the patient will feel light and may experience a pleasant feeling quite difficult to describe. If the bioplasmic body of the healer has a much lower rate of vibration than that of the patient, the patient may feel heaviness, discomfort, and sometimes pain. The bioplasmic body of the healer is usually more refined than that of the patient.

People who are heavy smokers have a coarser bioplasmic body. The bioplasmic body of a heavy smoker is filled with dirty brown spots. This brownish material partially clogs the nadis or meridians, and negatively affects the health of the smoker. The brown spots are located not only on the lungs but on other parts of the bioplasmic body, causing not only lung ailments but also other types of ailments. When a healer with a more refined bioplasmic body is contaminated by a heavy smoker, the healer would feel stickiness, heaviness and pain on the area being touched. It is very important that the healer be a nonsmoker or should give up smoking because instead of the patient becoming better, the patient might become worse, especially if the part being treated is quite delicate. To fully appreciate this, ask a heavy smoker to energize your arm and observe what happens.

I am not making any moral judgment on smokers. I am just pointing out that smoking has negative effects on the body. And that a pranic healer should not smoke because of the possible harmful effects on the patient. I know a few healers who smoke lightly, and have not reported any negative experience with their patients. But still it is better to avoid unnecessary risks. The dirty brownish matter can be transferred to another person. Just imagine what would happen to the patient if some dirty brownish matter were accidentally transferred to the eyes or heart of the patient.

Sometimes the patient may feel slight pain and heaviness on the part being energized if the healer is tired and has had an emotionally strenuous day. The healer should rest and resume healing the next day or when he or she feels better.

On rare occasions, the patient may have a very refined bioplasmic body or the rate of vibration of the patient's bioplasmic body is much higher than that of the healer. Such a patient, if treated by a healer whose bioplasmic body is coarser, would only experience more discomfort; in such a case, the patient should be treated by a healer whose bioplasmic body is as refined or more refined than that of the patient.

As a healer continues to practice healing, his or her bioplasmic body is gradually being cleansed and refined. The inner aura becomes brighter and denser and he or she becomes a more powerful healer.

Self-Healing

IN SELF-HEALING, the same basic principles of cleansing and energizing are used. There are several methods of healing oneself. You may use the manual approach, the pore breathing technique, the taoist technique, or the chakral breathing technique.

> After long hours at my desk translating Chinese texts, I sometimes felt very tired and nearly exhausted. But five minutes of these yogic breathing exercises would renew my strength and enable me to get on with my work. It cured my rheumatism and gave me instant relief not only when I caught cold but also when I contracted the dreaded Asian flu many years ago.[4]

MANUAL APPROACH

1) Do pranic breathing.

2) With the use of your hands, apply localized sweeping and energizing

---

[4]Charles Luk (Lu K'uan Yu), *The Secrets of Chinese Meditation* (York Beach, ME: Samuel Weiser, 1984).

on the chakra and part to be treated. Throw the diseased bioplasmic matter into the bioplasmic waste disposal unit. It is important that the "will" should be intensely applied.

3) The whole process should be continued until healing is complete or the condition has greatly improved.

PORE BREATHING TECHNIQUE

1) Do pranic breathing. Inhale and visualize prana or white light going into the pores of the affected part.

2) Retain your breath for a few seconds and visualize the grayish diseased matter becoming lighter or the affected parts becoming brighter.

3) Exhale and visualize the grayish diseased matter being expelled through the pores and through the health rays. Visualize the health rays being straightened. Straightening the health rays is very important since it is through the health rays that "used up" prana and diseased bioplasmic matter are expelled from the body.

4) Hold your breath for a few seconds and visualize the treated part as becoming brighter.

In pore breathing, you just simply inhale fresh prana through the pore and exhale the grayish diseased matter. Pore breathing is practiced by some students of ki kung or esoteric martial arts and by some students of hermetic science.

TAOIST TECHNIQUE OR TAOIST SIX HEALING SOUNDS

This Taoist healing technique is the same as the pore breathing technique except that specific sounds are shouted out for specific organs to facilitate the expelling of the diseased bioplasmic matter. The six healing sounds are:

Spleen: Hu (as in WHO)
Heart: Ho (as in WHOLE)

Lungs: Szu (as in SHUH)
Stomach: Hsi (as in SHIP)
Liver: Hsu (as in SHOE)
Kidneys: Ch'ui (as in JOY)

I am not so particular about the specific sound used for the specific organ. This Taoist self-healing technique is similar to practicing the martial arts. Every time the practitioner strikes and exhales, he shouts. What is important is the intention (or the will) to expel the diseased bioplasmic matter which is facilitated by shouting when exhaling.

CHAKRAL BREATHING TECHNIQUE

1) Do pranic breathing. Inhale slowly and concentrate on the affected chakra. Visualize the chakra drawing in or inhaling fresh prana. Hold your breath for a few seconds and visualize the prana being assimilated. Exhale slowly and visualize the chakra throwing out or exhaling the grayish dirty matter. Hold your breath for a few seconds and visualize the chakra becoming brighter and healthier. Repeat the process four times.

2) Do pranic breathing. Inhale slowly and concentrate on the affected organ. Visualize the chakra and the organ inhaling or drawing in prana. Visualize the prana as passing through the chakra, then to the affected organ. Hold your breath for a few seconds and visualize the chakra and the affected organ becoming brighter. Exhale slowly and visualize the grayish dirty matter being thrown out by the affected organ through the chakra. Hold your breath for a few seconds and visualize the chakra and the affected organ becoming brighter. Repeat the process until there is substantial relief. This technique is called chakral breathing.

Instead of exhaling slowly, the exhalation can be done forcefully and quickly with or without accompanied shouting. The exhalation is done through the mouth. Simultaneously, visualize the grayish diseased matter being thrown out of the affected organ through the chakra.

If you feel heaviness or pranic congestion on the chakra and in its organ or organs after doing chakral breathing, just inhale without willing prana to go into the chakra and its corresponding organ or organs. Exhale and visualize prana going out of the chakra and its corresponding organ or organs. Visualize the chakra becoming duller. Continue doing this until the condition normalizes.

Chakral breathing technique is very potent, and the relief is usually immediate for simple ailments. *Overdoing the chakral breathing technique may result in pranic congestion in the chakra and its corresponding organs. Overdoing it for a prolonged period of time will result in physical and psychological ailments.* The negative effect or effects are usually not felt immediately but are usually felt only after a few hours or after a day. This is just like having a big overdose of a potent drug. Chakral breathing should be practiced with moderation.

Caution should be taken when doing chakral breathing on the head chakras, heart chakra and eye chakras since their corresponding organs are quite delicate and could easily be congested. Chakral breathing should preferably not be done on the meng mein chakra, basic chakra and spleen chakra unless supervised by a competent teacher. Doing chakral breathing on these three chakras may result in severe pranic congestion in the entire body which may manifest as weakening of the body, high blood pressure or allergy throughout the body.

Pregnant women should not practice chakral breathing on the navel chakra, sex chakra, spleen chakra, meng mein chakra and basic chakra because it may adversely affect the unborn child.

GENERAL CLEANSING AND ENERGIZING

If your body is quite weak (or if infection is involved), then general cleansing and energizing should be applied. This is necessary not only to energize yourself but also to seal the holes in the outer aura and to partially disentangle the health rays. There are several ways that you can do this.

Method 1: Pranic Breathing

Diffuse or scatter your consciousness to all parts of your body. Do pranic breathing for ten cycles. Inhale slowly. Will and feel prana going into all parts of your body. Exhale slowly and visualize grayish diseased matter being expelled from all parts of the body. Visualize the health rays as being straight. After doing pranic breathing for about ten breathing cycles, meditate on your navel for about ten minutes and simultaneously do pranic breathing before ending the session. When you become proficient, you will feel pranic energy going into all parts of your body.

Method 2: Visualization Approach

Do pranic breathing. Visualize yourself or another person applying general sweeping, localized sweeping and energizing with prana to your body. Visualize and will your body becoming brighter, the health rays becoming disentangled, and the outer aura brighter. Be sure to dispose of the dirty diseased bioplasmic matter.

Method 3: Meditation on the White Light

This method of general cleansing and energizing is usually called meditation on the white light or meditation on the middle pillar. The middle pillar technique has been used by various oriental and occidental esoteric schools. This technique is divided into two parts. The first part deals with general cleansing and energizing. The second part deals with the circulation of prana.

Part I: General Cleansing and Energizing

1) Do pranic breathing and simultaneously visualize a ball of intense bright light above the crown.

2) Visualize a stream of light coming down from the ball to the crown, then gradually down to the feet. Visualize the white light cleansing and energizing all the major chakras, all the important organs, the spine, and the bones in the body.

3) Visualize the white light coming out of the feet and flushing out all the grayish diseased matter. Repeat the process three times.

4) Visualize a brilliant ball of light at the bottom of the feet. Draw in earth prana in the form of a stream of light from this brilliant ball of light. Inhale and draw in the prana through the sole chakras up to the head. Exhale and let the prana sprinkle out of the crown chakra. Repeat this three times.

Part 2: *Circulating Prana*

1) Visualize prana circulating from the bottom of the feet, up to the back of the body, up to the head, down to the face, to the front of the body, then to the feet. Circulate prana from back to front three times.

2) Reverse the circulation and circulate prana from front to back. Circulate three times.

3) Circulate prana from left to right three times and from right to left three times. The purpose of circulating prana is to evenly distribute prana throughout the body and to prevent pranic congestion in certain parts of the body.

This meditation can be used daily to improve and maintain your health. It is also used by some esoteric students before engaging in activities that require a lot of prana. You may perform this meditation before healing a large number of people. Though there are many variations of this meditation, the one presented here is simplified and easy to perform.

Once you become proficient in this meditation, some of you will literally feel your body tingle and will feel a strong current moving within and outside your body.

You may also use the excess prana generated to produce "synthetic ki" or navel ki by concentrating on the navel chakra for about ten minutes. Store the "synthetic ki" in the two secondary navel chakras located two inches below the navel. This is done by simply concentrating on two inches below the navel for about three to five minutes. Pranic breathing should be done simultaneously with the preceding instructions.

Each of the secondary navel chakras has a big flexible meridian that is used for storing navel ki. In short, the two secondary navel chakras are warehouses for the "synthetic ki." The two secondary navel chakras are called *ki hai*, which means "ocean of ki" because these minor chakras are filled with "synthetic ki." It must be repeated that "synthetic ki" or navel ki is different from prana. The "synthetic ki" is synthesized by the navel chakra and may appear as milky white, whitish red, golden yellow, and other colors. The "synthetic ki" varies in size and in density. Ordinary persons have very little "synthetic ki" compared to spiritual aspirants and practitioners of ki kung.

It would be advisable for you to learn to meditate on the white light and practice it every day. It makes your bioplasmic body cleaner, brighter, and denser, thereby making you a better healer.

PHYSICAL EXERCISES

Physical exercise plays a vital role in self-healing and in maintaining health. Physical exercises in the form of warmup exercises, dancing, sports, hatha yoga, martial arts or tai chi promote circulation of prana in the body and facilitate the drawing in of fresh prana and the expelling of used-up prana or diseased bioplasmic matter. This is seen clairvoyantly as white fresh prana being drawn in and grayish diseased matter being thrown out when one is exercising. It is better if pranic breathing is done when exercising. There are specific physical exercises in hatha yoga and Taoist yoga to treat specific ailments. The type of exercise can easily be determined by observing and analyzing which part of the body is being moved, bent, compressed or stretched by a specific pose or exercise and the particular chakra located on that part affected by the exercise.

As a matter of fact, you can develop your own exercises or techniques to clean and energize a specific chakra. All you have to do is invent certain motions that would move, bend, compress and stretch that part of the body where the specific chakra is located. Physical exercises also facilitate the assimilation of prana after pranic treatment. A good exercise should consist of a short series of motions that would clean and energize all the major chakras and all the minor chakras on the arms and legs.

HOLISTIC APPROACH TO SELF-HEALING

1) Do physical exercise for five to ten minutes.

2) Apply pranic self healing.

3) Do physical exercise on the treated chakra and organ for a few minutes to facilitate the assimilation of prana by the body.

4) Drink energized water or water that has been exposed to the sun.

5) Rest and recuperate under a big tree (or a big pine tree) to absorb prana from the tree and the ground.

6) Take medication. Faster healing is obtained by simultaneously treating the bioplasmic body and the visible physical body, rather than treating the visible physical body alone or the bioplasmic body alone. As stated

in the earlier chapter, the treatment should preferably be holistic or integrated.

7) For severe ailments, consult a reputable pranic healer and a reputable medical doctor.

Eating proper food, drinking enough water, proper breathing, sufficient physical exercise, living a moderate lifestyle, having a calm disposition, and a clear decisive mind would greatly contribute and help maintain physical, emotional and mental wellbeing.

PROBLEMS ENCOUNTERED IN SELF-HEALING

Some healers may find it difficult to heal themselves. This could be due to several possible factors. For example, the body of the healer may have become very weak and in pain, thereby making concentration and utilization of the will difficult. The healer may be good at projecting prana but may have little practice in self-healing. The healer is either too tired or weak or doesn't care enough, or the healer simply prefers to rest and be healed by another healer.

Sometimes the ailment requires treatment using other supplementary or more appropriate forms of healing combined with pranic healing. On rare occasions, healing oneself of a serious ailment is not possible due to karmic factors or negative karma.

Many healers sometimes find it difficult to heal themselves and I am no exception. I do not hesitate to take medication whenever necessary, consult a medical doctor, get an acupressure massage or seek the help of another healer when I do not feel well. There are also times when I prefer to rest and let the other healer do the healing.

Karma

Some serious ailments are due to negative deeds, thoughts, and feelings in the present and past lives of patients. This is called *negative karma*. But not all serious ailments are due to negative karma. No pranic healer should ever turn away a patient just because he or she thinks the ailment may be due to negative karma! Very few clairvoyants can actually see with great accuracy into the past karma of a patient. Even if it is negative karma, you are not in a position to know when the negative karma has been fully worked out; therefore the patient is entitled to be healed. If the ailment is due to negative karma and it has not been worked out, then no amount of treatment can heal the patient. So the healer can in no way interfere with the negative karma of the patient.

For instance, I was approached by a woman with a seriously injured right leg. The leg was quite painful from the hip down to the foot. It was almost impossible for the patient to move the right hip or knee without causing intense pain. Pranic healing was applied for about thirty minutes. The pain was greatly reduced. She was able to partially bend her knee and move her hip without any pain. On the day she was scheduled to have her second treatment, she was involved in three freak accidents involving her right leg. These caused intense suffering, making it very difficult for her to visit me. The patient has not returned for further treatment ever since. For these three "accidents" to occur in a matter of few hours is probably a case of negative karma. (For more information on karma, please refer to reading materials from Edgar Cayce, Astara, theosophy, agni yoga, Rosicrucian, and other esoteric groups.)

Karma, in its broadest sense, means that what you sow is what you reap, or what you give is what you receive (Galatians 6:7). It means the law of cause and effect as applied to an individual or a group of individuals, such as a family, a corporation or a nation.

The law of karma, when applied positively, manifests as the positive golden rule: "do unto others what you would have others do unto you." The golden rule can be applied to get what you want or desire. If you want to be prosperous, then you must give and practice charity. If you want cordiality and harmony, then you should be cordial and courteous to others.

The law of karma can be used to avoid undesirable things or events when it is applied as a "negative" golden rule, which is "do not do unto others what you do not want others to do unto you." If you do not want to be cheated or swindled, then treat others honestly and fairly. If you have worked out most of your negative karma and have not done anybody any harm, then you have nothing to fear. Nothing can harm you. The law of karma is unbreakable. This is the meaning behind the statement that "my righteousness is my shield." Literally, nothing can harm such a person. A thousand or million people may fall beside this person but not even a single strand of hair will be touched!

The golden rule will produce harmony and prosperity in your life and protect you from the vicissitudes of life. If the golden rule could be applied by most people and by most nations, it would bring about world peace! The law of karma is also the basis of the command given by Jesus "to love your enemy." Returning hate with hate, anger with anger, spite with spite, malicious injury with more malicious injury only makes things worse. There is no end to these. What you give is what you receive! To return hate with hate will only bring chaos, but to return hate with kindness and love will inevitably result in harmony and peace. It is, indeed, a pity that after almost two thousand years, the teachings of Christ are only given lip service and not put into action by the majority of His followers. The command "to love your enemy" was not only taught by Christ but was also taught by Gautama Buddha and other religious teachers.

> So long as an evil deed has not karmically matured, the fool thinks his deed to be sweet as honey. But, when his evil deed karmically matures, he falls into untold misery.
>
> —*Dhammapada* (Wisdom of the Buddha)

The more he gives to others, the more he has.

> —Lao Tsu
> *Tao Te Ching*

> Each man, by the action of unerring karma, receives in exact measure all that is due, all that he deserves, neither more nor less. Not one benevolent or evil action, trifling as it may be, as secretly as it may done, escapes the precisely balanced scale of karma.[5]
>
> —Helena Roerich
> *Foundations of Buddhism*

SUGGESTED ETHICAL GUIDELINES

1) It is your duty as a healer to try your best to heal and alleviate the condition of patients.

2) The healer is entitled to charge a reasonable rate for services. The healer should avoid charging excessive fees that would unduly burden the patient.

---

[5]Helena Roerich, *Foundations of Buddhism* (New York: Agni Yoga Society, 1971).

3) Under no circumstances should a healer turn away or neglect a patient due to poverty or inability of the patient to pay.

4) The healer should withhold any information concerning the case of patients to others if the disclosure of such information will or may cause embarrassment to the patient.

5) Under no circumstances should a healer take sexual advantage of patients. Whenever possible or permissible, healing should be done in the open or in front of others. Healing in a closed room with the healer and patient alone should, as much as possible, be avoided and minimized.

Most patients are quite gullible or easily influenced. This is due to two factors: the ability of the healer to produce amazing results; and that some patients do not know what to expect or what will be required of them during pranic healing.

6) Under no circumstances should you, as a healer misuse your power. Power or the ability to manipulate invisible subtle energies is neither good nor bad. Power is good when used constructively, and bad when used for destruction. It becomes bad when there is evil intention and misapplication of power.

TERMINOLOGY

Pranic healing or ki healing has been called by many names, such as magnetic healing, faith healing, psychic healing, and the laying on of hands. Unfortunately, these names are inaccurate and misleading. The use of these names would only make accurate and deeper study difficult if not impossible.

There is nothing magnetic about the hands. The left hand is not negative or receptive nor is the right hand positive or projective. Both hands or hand chakras are capable of absorbing and projecting prana. It is just a matter of intention, or willing which hand chakra to predominantly absorb and which one to predominantly project. The energy or prana projected is not magnetic, but rather vitalizing and strengthening. This is why the use of the term magnetic healing for pranic healing is inaccurate. This does not in any way minimize the effectivity of magnetic healing.

The terms psychic healing, faith healing, laying on of hands, etc., are too broad and could mean and imply many things to different people.

Therefore, it is not advisable to use these terms loosely. For example, the laying on of hands describes to a certain extent only the outward acts but does not explain or describe what is happening inwardly or invisibly. Therefore, it would give the misconception that the act of laying on of hands causes the healing. It is actually the involuntary or deliberate projection of prana (vital energy) from the hand to the affected part (and in some cases the involuntary absorption of the diseased bioplasmic matter by the hand into the body of the healer) that causes the healing.

Another possible term that could be used to describe pranic healing would be *bioplasmic healing*, since it is by healing the bioplasmic body that the visible physical body is correspondingly healed.

INVOCATIVE PRANIC HEALING

It is a common practice by some pranic healers to make an invocation or to say a prayer before starting to heal. The invocation may be directed to God, to divine beings, or to one's spiritual guides. There are some invocative pranic healers who may not understand the principles and the mechanics behind the healing process. They just simply feel a tremendous power flowing into their bodies causing the body to vibrate and become warm. Some invocative healers may not be so sensitive that they feel the flow of energy into their bodies. This does not in any way alter the fact that their bodies are being used as channels for healing energy. There are also cases where the inflowing of healing power triggers temporarily the clairvoyant faculty of the healers. Those who practice invocative pranic healing are usually called faith healers or charismatic healers. See figure 40 on page 155.

In invocative healing you are invoking two things: the healing energy and the mighty invisible spiritual beings or healing angels. These mighty spiritual beings or healing angels are the ones manipulating and controlling the healing energy and the bioplasmic body of the patients, thereby ensuring the safety of the patients. The invocative pranic healer should maintain a receptive attitude in order to receive intuitive guidance or instruction. For healers who are quite willful, they should be careful when practicing invocative pranic healing since there is the danger of overenergizing the patient.

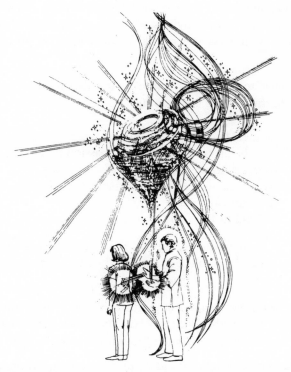

Figure 40. Pranic invocative healing—the downpouring of spiritual healing energy.

If it is time for the patient to leave his or her body, the healing angels will not appear. The healer will usually be intuitively aware that there is no response.

Although some invocative pranic healers or faith healers may not be knowledgeable about pranic healing, this does not in any way diminish their potency and effectivity. Some of these healers can heal at a very fast rate and for many hours without getting tired. Even advanced pranic healers would find it difficult to duplicate what invocative pranic healers are capable of doing.

If you intend to go into healing by prayer or invocative pranic healing, then it is advisable that you meditate and pray regularly and request the Lord to make you His instrument for healing.

The invocative healing techniques given below are applicable to all persons of any religious denomination. They are quite potent and effective. One does not have to be religious for it to work; just believe in God and trust that with God everything is possible! The procedure is as follows:

1) Pray for a few minutes any religious prayer that you are used to. Then mentally recite the healing invocation:

> Lord, make me Thy healing instrument.
> Let my entire being be filled with compassion for
>   others who are suffering.
> Lord, let Your healing and regenerating power flow
>   through this body.
> With thanks and in full faith!

The invocation should be repeated two times with intense concentration and full conviction. It should be done with humility, sincerity, and reverence.

2) For those with background in pranic healing, apply pranic treatment on the patient. Thank the Lord for His Divine Blessing after you have finished the treatment. Request the patient to thank the Lord.

3) For those with no background in pranic healing, simply place your hand on the affected area or on the crown chakra or on the ajna chakra. Then mentally recite and invoke:

> Father,
> Thank you for healing this patient!
> In full faith, so be it!

It is important to maintain the proper attitude that you are only a divine healing channel. Continue your invocation and concentrating on the center of your palm until you feel that the patient will be all right. Be in tune for intuitive instructions. Before ending the treatment, the healer and the patient should give thanks to the Lord.

For simple ailments, the cure is usually instantaneous. For more severe ailments, the relief is fast but complete recovery may require several treatments. Treatment has to be given several times a week depending upon the needs of the patient. Invocative healing can be applied to a group of patients by a healer or it can be done by a group of invocative healers on a patient.

When I do healing, I prefer to use a simpler and shorter invocation:

Father, thank you for making me Thy healing
instrument. In full faith!

I mentally recite the above invocation two to three times.

Negative karma sometimes can be neutralized through divine intercession. For students who intend to go full time into healing and who want to practice invocative pranic healing, it is important that they should undergo a period of refining or improving their character. The downpouring of the healing energy together with the spiritual energy magnifies many times the positive and negative characteristics of the healer, hence, the necessity for self-purification through the daily practice of inner reflection. Also, a person with refined or higher vibration tends to attract entities with similar or higher vibrations while a person with gross or lower vibrations or characteristics tends to attract undesirable entities with similar low vibrations.

Spiritual chanting, singing and dancing are other forms of invocative healing. This type of invocative healing is universal and is used by some Christians, Sufis and people of other religious faiths.

ASSIGNING HEALING ANGELS

After treatment, it is better to request the Lord to assign a healing angel to remain with each patient suffering from severe ailments in order to further accelerate the healing process. The patient should be instructed to be more receptive by invoking the Lord's blessing several times a day. Receptiveness of the patient will make the work of the healing angel a lot easier. The healer can request a healing angel to be assigned to the patient by mentally reciting this prayer:

Lord, thank you for assigning a healing
angel to remain with the patient until he is
completely cured. In full faith. So be it!

It is important that the invocation be done with humility, sincerity, and reverence.

PRINCIPLE OF DIVERSION OR RELEASING

One day, I had a severe headache. Instead of healing myself or asking a friend to heal me, I decided to experiment. What would happen if I concentrated fully on listening to soothing music? What would happen to my bioplasmic body and to the diseased bioplasmic matter?

Based on a clairvoyant's observation, it was noted that when I started to concentrate fully on the music, the grayish diseased matter gradually and slowly started to thin out or become lighter, even to the extent of almost disappearing. After five to ten minutes, I got up and tried to feel the condition of my head. There was a slight reduction in pain. It was also noted that when my attention was withdrawn from the music and directed to the head area, the head area suddenly became more grayish. The final condition, however, was much lighter than when the experiment started. There are several possible explanations to what happened:

1) Relaxing the mind and the body facilitates the body to heal itself.

2) Since the bioplasmic body is easily affected by mind and emotion, then anything that has a positive effect on the mind must have some positive effect on the bioplasmic body.

3) By diverting the attention to something that is pleasant or harmonious, the diseased bioplasmic matter was released, or the hold was loosened; thereby allowing the body to heal itself more effectively. This is why the grayish matter became thinner or lighter. It seems that when attention is focused on the pain, this tends to hold together the diseased bioplasmic matter, thereby hindering the healing process.

4) By concentrating again on the affected part, the diseased bioplasmic matter was drawn back. That is why the affected part became grayish again.

I observed that if I am focusing on the pain and trying to remove it, I find it more difficult to heal myself. But if I just ignore the pain and concentrate fully on what I am visualizing, the rate of healing is very fast.

The principle of diversion or releasing is also applicable in healing others. When some patients become so engrossed with the strange movements of the healer, their concentration on the pain they are experiencing is temporarily distracted, thereby facilitating the healing process. At times when the attention of the patient is so focused on the pain, or the discomfort is so intense, then it would be very helpful to ask the patient to concentrate on soothing music or on a very nice picture. Letting the patient listen to soothing music through earphones would undoubtedly be even more effective.

> People have little idea how much they increase the potency of the disease by the constantly directed thought which they expend upon it [by thinking too much about the ailment], and the attention they pay to that area wherein the trouble is located.[6]

TEACHING PATIENTS HOW TO HEAL THEMSELVES

It is advisable for severely sick patients to be taught pranic self-healing even if they are treated by conventional methods or by pranic healing. They can be taught certain physical exercises that will clean and energize the affected chakra and organ. Pore breathing or the Taoist healing technique can also be taught. The patients should be supervised regularly in order to correct possible pranic congestion due to pore breathing.

The patients should be instructed to drink energized water and to recuperate under a big tree or a big pine tree. Some patients go even to the extent of embracing a big tree. Patients should also engage in enjoyable and productive activities rather than brood over their predicaments or ailments. See figure 41 on page 160.

Patients who are religious can pray regularly and request the Lord to make them whole and perfect again. There are, however, some people who are not comfortable with prayer, or who don't belong to any particular religious faith. These patients can learn to work with visualization in order to contact their spiritual guides. To do this, they should first relax and visualize themselves in a beautiful garden. In that garden, they meet beings of light. They humbly request help and healing from these beings of light. Patients should visualize a pool of water filled with light, and visualize themselves immersed in that pool. By washing in the pool of water and light, the entire body is cleansed and energized. At the end of such a visualization, the patient should give thanks for help and healing.

The visualizations do not have to be clear—the patient doesn't have to actually see these beings of light. What is important during such sessions

---

[6]Alice Bailey, *Esoteric Healing* (New York: Lucis Publishing, 1977).

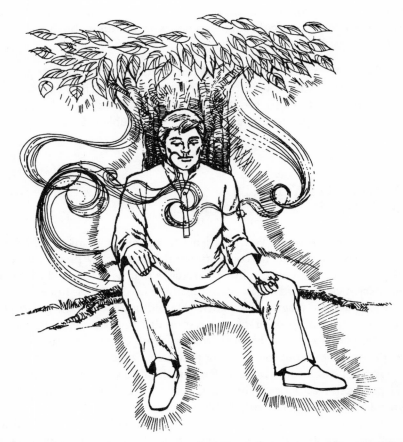

Figure 41. Resting under a tree to absorb pranic energy from the tree and the ground. Both healers and patients can use this technique.

is that the patient divert his or her attention away from the ailment or discomfort, thereby giving the body a greater opportunity to heal itself. Prayer and visualization are both good techniques to enhance self-healing. Although there is no guarantee that most terminal patients will be healed, their conditions will be improved to a certain degree and the pain will be greatly alleviated. Visualization and prayer are both excellent tools because they can help people to heal themselves or they can help people go within and make peace with death."

LEVEL THREE: ABSENT HEALING

The planetary-etheric body is whole, unbroken and continuous; of this etheric body, those of the healer and of the patient are integral, intrinsic parts. . . . The channels of relationship can be conductors of many different types of energy, transmitted by the healer to the patient.

—Alice Bailey
Esoteric Healing

Prana [vital energy] colored by the thought of the sender may be projected to persons at a distance, who are willing to receive it, and the healing can be done this way.

—Yogi Ramacharaka
The Science of Psychic Healing

Energy follows thought.

—An Esoteric Maxim

9

Distant Pranic Healing

THE MECHANISM behind distant healing is similar to that of the telephone. The healer and the patient are linked because their etheric bodies are parts of earth's etheric body. When the healer focuses his attention on the patient, he or she can remove diseased etheric matter and project prana (vital energy) to the patient since energy follows thought. Distant pranic healing is similar to close-ranged pranic healing. The only difference is that in distant pranic healing, the psychic faculty of the healer has to be developed or sharpened further through regular practice for greater accuracy. Those of you who have been healing or experimenting on healing may have developed the skill to sense what part is wrong with the patient even without scanning. Some may have even developed the psychic sense to feel or even see vaguely the degree of healthiness of an organ that is being energized. The unfolding or gradual development of the psychic faculty is a natural by-product in healing. It is advisable that before you try distant pranic healing, you should have at least gained proficiency in intermediate pranic healing.

DISTANT SCANNING

The ability to scan a patient at a distance is something that has to be gradually developed through regular practice. In order to learn this, you need to do the following:

1) Every time a patient comes to you for healing, don't scan the patient with your hands and don't interview him or her immediately.

2) Let your patient sit in front of you. Close your eyes and try to psychically see and scan the bioplasmic body and visible physical body of your patient. Look at the chakras from the crown down to the feet. Pay special attention to the major chakras. Are the chakras bright, grayish, muddy red or black? Try to scan them also. Are they thick or thin or just normal? You may imagine you are scanning with your hands. Look and scan the important organs from top to bottom. Do they look and feel good? Do they look too reddish or do they look bluish? Look and feel the spine from top to bottom. Do you see or feel any obstruction or slight dislocation? You do not have to see clearly or very lucidly in order to be accurate. Being able to see or scan vaguely would be good enough. Relax; do it slowly but thoroughly. The patient will not mind waiting for a few minutes.

3) Open your eyes. Get up and scan the patient thoroughly.

4) Interview the patient. Evaluate the condition of the patient and compare it with the findings from your psychic scan.

It is possible that you will achieve some degree of accuracy even on the first try. Continue practicing until you become not only relatively accurate but very accurate. This may require at least several months of regular practice. Proper and effective treatment depends upon accurate scanning.

Try actual distant diagnosis and scanning first on patients you have treated before. Then gradually try it on patients whom you have never met. Get a picture of the patient to help you establish a contact with him or her.

DISTANT CLEANSING AND ENERGIZING

Distant cleansing and energizing are a lot easier and faster to learn. There are two methods that you can use:

Method 1

1) Do pranic breathing. Visualize the patient in front of you. Do not visualize the patient as very far from you since this would tend to condition your mind that the entire endeavor is very difficult.

2) Visualize or imagine that you are applying general and localized sweeping on the parts to be treated. Dispose of the diseased bioplasmic matter by visualizing a fire or a ball of light as bright as the sun beside you and the diseased matter being thrown into it. Continue cleansing until the treated parts look brighter.

3) Energize the affected chakras and parts to be treated. Continue energizing until the treated parts look quite bright and healthy or until you feel the treated parts have enough prana. You just simply feel the patient has enough prana or the treated part is already full and is no longer absorbing prana.

4) Get up and open your eyes. Scan the patient to determine whether he or she has been properly treated. If not, repeat the entire process until the treated parts have substantially improved. Wash your hands after the treatment.

Method 2

1) Let the patient sit in front of you and close your eyes.

2) Visualize a brilliant ball of light on top of the patient. Visualize a stream of white light washing the head area and gradually going down and cleansing the entire body. Gather the diseased bioplasmic matter and dispose of it properly.

3) Visualize the grayish matter in the affected part as becoming less dense and lighter. Will it to come out or see it as floating out.

4) The diseased bioplasmic matter can be disposed of by willing it to disintegrate immediately or by visualizing the grayish matter as gradually thinning out, or you can simply visualize a fire and throw the diseased bioplasmic matter into it.

5) Energize the affected parts. This is done by visualizing a ball of light (pranic ball) being formed and projecting it to the affected part.

6) Open your eyes and rescan the patient. Give further treatment if required.

The difference between Method 1 and Method 2 is that in Method 1, prana is being drawn into the body of the healer before projecting it to the patient. In Method 2, prana is drawn from the surroundings and projected directly to the patient without passing through the body of the healer. You can also combine Method 1 and Method 2.

After you have become proficient, you can try healing familiar patients at a distance. Then you can gradually try new patients.

REFERENCES AND SUGGESTED READING

Babbit, Edwin. *The Principles of Light and Color: The Healing Power of Color*. Secaucus, NJ: Citadel Press, Reprint, 1967.

Bardon, Franz. A. Radspieler, trans. *Initiation Into Hermetics*. Wuppertal, W. Germany: Dieter Rüggeberg, 1956.

Blofeld, John. *Gateway To Wisdom: Taoist and Buddhist Contemplative and Healing Yogas Adapted for Western Students*. Boston, MA: Shambhala, 1913.

Burke, Abbot George. *Magnetic Therapy*. Oklahoma City, OK: Saint George Press, 1980.

Chia, Mantak. *Awaken Healing Energy Through the Tao*. Santa Fe, NM: Aurora Press, 1983.

Clark, Linda and Marine, Yvonne. *Health, Youth and Beauty Through Color Breathing*. Millbrae, CA: Celestial Arts, 1976.

Harner, Michael. *The Way of the Shaman: A Guide to Power and Healing*. New York: Bantam Books, 1980.

Hunt, Roland. *The Seven Keys to Colour Healing*. Saffron Walden, England: C. W. Daniel, 1971.

Hwa, Jou Tsung. *The Tao of Meditation: Way to Enlightenment*. Piscataway, NJ: Tai Chi Foundation, 1983.

Karp, Rebecca Ann. *Edgar Cayce: Encyclopedia of Healing*. New York: Warner Books, 1986.

Krieger, Dolores, Ph.D. *The Therapeutic Touch*. Englewood Cliffs, NJ: Prentice-Hall, 1979.

Long, Max Freedom. *The Secret Science at Work*. Marina del Rey, CA: DeVorss, 1953.

Ramacharaka, Yogi. *The Science of Psychic Healing.* Homewood, IL: Yoga Publishing Society, 1909.

Regardie, Israel. *The Art of True Healing.* Phoenix, AZ: Falcon Press, 1937.

Wallace, Amy and Henkin, Bill. *The Psychic Healing Book.* Berkeley, CA: Wingbow Press, 1978.

Wu, K. H., ed., Ping, Lheng, trans. *Therapeutic Breathing Exercises.* Hong Kong: Hai Feng Publishing, 1984.

Yu, Lu K'uan. *The Secret of Chinese Meditation.* York Beach, ME: Samuel Weiser, 1964; and London: Rider & Co., 1964.

LEVEL FOUR: ADVANCED PRANIC HEALING

A professor visited a Roshi (Zen master) to learn about Zen. The professor was more interested in talking and trying to impress the Zen master than in learning. The Roshi invited the professor for a drink and poured tea into the professor's cup and continued pouring until it was overflowing. The professor alarmingly said, "the cup is full and cannot receive more!" The Zen master calmly replied, "You are full of preconceived ideas and opinions. To learn, you must empty your cup!" The professor respectfully bowed to the Roshi and remained silent.

—A Popular Zen Story

Miracles are fantastic events which utilize hidden laws of nature that most people are not aware of. Miracles do not break the laws of nature, they are actually based on them!

—C.K.S.

Color Pranic Healing

THIS CHAPTER is predominantly based on the instructions given me by my teacher, Mei Ling, who is one of my mentors in esoteric studies. Some of the concepts and techniques are new and are different from other books on color healing. Instructions on the art of instantaneous healing of fresh wounds are given in this chapter. Many of the advanced techniques should be practiced preferably by experienced pranic healers, and not by beginners.

Advanced pranic healing uses pranic color healing and chakral pranic healing to produce very rapid healing and to cure difficult ailments.

Air prana, solar prana and ground prana are made of white or general prana. Air and ground pranas are calld vitality globules in esoteric parlance because when seen clairvoyantly or by a person with slightly more sensitive eyes, they appear as small spheres or globules of light. Vitality globules come in different sizes. Some contain more units of white prana and some contain less.

Ground vitality globules interpenetrate the ground and extend several inches away from it. They are denser or more closely-packed and usually bigger than air vitality globules. Some of the bigger air vitality globules can be easily seen just by staring at the sky for a few minutes, especially just before sunset. You do not need to be a clairvoyant to be able to see air vitality globules. A lot of you will be able to see them in a few sessions.

Also, with more practice you will be able to see ground vitality globules just a few inches away from the ground.

COLOR PRANAS

Vitality globules (conglomerations of units of white prana) are absorbed by the chakras where they are digested and broken down to their components. When white prana is digested, it produces six types of color pranas that correspond to the colors of the rainbow. A substantial amount of air prana is absorbed directly by the spleen chakra (front and back). The air prana is broken down to different color pranas and distributed to the other chakras. Ground prana is absorbed through the sole chakras. A portion of the ground prana is directed upward to the spine and other chakras, while a large portion is directed to the perineum minor chakra, to the navel chakra, then to the spleen chakra, where it is broken down and distributed to the other chakras. All these take place automatically or at a subconscious level.

White prana is composed of red, orange, yellow, green, blue, and violet pranas. Of the six color pranas, red, blue, and green pranas are most frequently used in healing. The properties of each of the six color pranas and their applications are listed below.

Red Prana

Strengthening (vitalizing and vigorous)
Warm
Distributive (improves circulation)
Constructive—rapid tissue or cellular repair
Sustains the visible physical body
Vitalizes the blood, tissues and skeletal system of the body.
Stimulating and activating

Red Prana Applications:
Internal and external wounds
Broken bones
Allergy

Sluggish or weakened organs or parts
General tiredness or weakening
Paralysis
Reviving unconscious patients
Reviving or prolonging the life of dying patients
Measles

Orange Prana

Expelling
Eliminative
Decongesting
Cleansing
Loosening (loosens diseased bioplasmic matter)
Melting
Extracting or abstracting
Splitting, exploding and destructive

Orange Prana Applications:
All ailments related to expelling or elimination of waste, germs, toxins and diseased bioplasmic matter.
Kidney and bladder ailments
Constipation
Menstrual problems
Removing blood clots
Arthritis
Cysts
Colds, coughs and lung problems

Orange prana has a very potent effect; therefore, it should be avoided in treating delicate organs like the eyes, the brain, and the heart. Intense energizing with orange prana on delicate organs may cause serious damage such as detached retina or hemorrhage of the brain. Orange prana should not be used on patients suffering from appendicitis because it may accelerate the rupture of the inflamed appendix. Orange prana is also used to facilitate the abstraction of consciousness of a dying patient.

Green Prana

Breaking down
Digestive
Decongesting
Detoxifying
Disinfecting
Dissolving
Loosening of diseased bioplasmic matter

Green Prana Applications:
Breaking down blood clots
Disinfectant
Colds
Fevers
Used in localized cleansing for decongesting and loosening stubborn diseased bioplasmic matter.

Orange or green prana is usually used in decongesting and cleansing a diseased part by loosening the diseased bioplasmic matter. After being loosened, the diseased bioplasmic matter is removed by localized sweeping and then the affected part is energized. The loosening and expelling of the diseased bioplasmic matter by orange or green prana would enable fresh prana to enter the affected part, thereby restoring health to that part.

Green prana is milder and safer than orange prana. When internal organs are to be energized with orange prana, it is advisable to use green prana first as a safety precaution before projecting orange prana.

Light green prana should be used first before energizing with more potent pranas such as orange, red and violet. This is done as a precautionary measure to avoid possible harm or damage on the patient. Energizing first with light green prana and then with light orange prana is very effective in decongesting, expelling and cleansing physically and bioplasmically the part being treated. Please, note the sequence. Light green prana is used first before light orange prana and not orange prana first nor both simultaneously. When light orange-green prana is projected or when both orange prana and green prana are projected simultaneously, the effects of these pranas are multiplied several times; therefore, the effect is destructive to a certain degree. When the darker shades of green and orange pranas are used, the effect is quite destructive, hence they are used in treating tumors. For a more potent effect, dark orange-green prana is used. (Blue prana would be used first in order to localize the disintegrating effect of the projected pranic energy on the affected part.)

Yellow Prana

Cohesion or cementing
Assimilating, multiplying and growth
Stimulating effect on the nerves
Initiating or starter

Yellow Prana Applications:
Wounds
Fractured bones
Skin problems
Cellular repairs

Blue Prana

Strong disinfectant
Inhibiting
Localizing and contracting
Soothing and mild anaesthetic
Cooling
Pliability or flexibility

Blue Prana Applications:
Ailments due to infection
Removing pain
Inflammation
Inhibit chakras, organs and motor action
Rest and sleep inducing
Stop bleeding
Fever

I experimented with color on a paralytic person. Treatment was first given to the brain, then to the right arm. Light blue prana was directed to the affected right arm for several minutes. As a result, the patient had greater difficulty in raising his right arm. When light red prana was directed to the affected area, the patient was able to move his right arm with greater ease. The next day there was even greater improvement. This shows that blue prana has an inhibiting effect while red prana has strengthening and stimulating effects.

Violet Prana

Violet prana has the properties of all the other five pranas and is very potent. It is used on severe types of ailments. It is usually not used on mild ailments. Light violet or green-violet prana is used for the rapid healing of partially damaged internal organs like severe gastric ulcers. Light violet prana is also used to treat severe infection, such as syphilis and pneumonia.

• • •

Through clairvoyant observation, the indigo color is normally not found in any of the chakras and in any part of the bioplasmic body; that is why only six types of color pranas are described in this chapter.

The effect of color prana is qualified and enhanced by the intention of the healer. For instance, blue prana can be used to inhibit a chakra or an organ by forming a strong intention to inhibit when projecting it.

Using color prana instead of white prana is just like approaching a specialist instead of a general practitioner. Color prana is more specialized and more potent than white prana. More visualization skills are needed in the use of color prana. I usually use a safer technique; I combine color prana of a lighter shade with white prana. I usually visualize the projected prana as luminous white at the core with a tinge of color prana on the periphery. For example, you can visualize the projected prana as brilliant or dazzling white at the core and with light red on the periphery to strengthen an organ. The potency of the color is diluted, thereby making it safer. White prana is the harmonizing prana. It is harmonizing in the sense that it provides other color pranas required in healing and redistributes excess color pranas required in healing and redistributes excess color pranas in the treated area to other parts of the body. Sometimes you can use undiluted light color prana or darker color prana for more potent effects.

When in doubt as to what color prana to use, just use white prana. I usually use white prana on infants, very young children, and on old patients. On certain occasions when white prana is not sufficiently effective, then color prana can be used. For instance, an allergy can be alleviated by using white or color pranas. But there are certain types of allergy that can only be relieved by using red prana. Using white prana or other color pranas will not produce any substantial effect on severe types of allergy.

To students or practitioners of color healing, the properties or qualities of green, yellow, and orange pranas may seem strange or doubtful. This was also my initial reaction but further study and experiments showed that these are correct. By experimenting on color pranas and studying the pranas contained in the chakras and the organs controlled and energized by the corresponding chakras, it is possible to deduce and verify the correctness of the properties or qualities of the different types of color prana.

CHAKRAS AND COLORS

The major chakras are three to four inches in diameter. More advanced yogis have major chakras that are five to six inches in diameter and are brighter and more refined. The major chakras control and energize the whole physical body and also control and affect one's psychological and spiritual conditions.

The *basic chakra* has four petals and contains red and orange pranas. The red prana from the basic chakra is used for energizing and strengthening the entire visible physical body—muscles, bones, blood, adrenal glands, sex organs, internal organs, general vitality, body heat—and the growth rate of infants and children. The quality of blood produced is influenced by the basic chakra. This chakra is very important and will be used very often in advanced pranic healing. Malfunctioning of this chakra may manifest as allergy, low vitality, cancer, sexual ailment, growth problem and also psychological disorders. *The basic chakra is the center of self-survival or self-preservation.* Some people whose basic chakras are underactive tend to be impractical, unrealistic or in some severe cases, they tend to be completely out of touch with reality. Persons with suicidal inclination tend to have weak and underactive basic chakras.

The *sex chakra* has six petals and contains red and orange pranas. This chakra contains red prana of two different shades. It controls and energizes the sex organs and the bladder. The sex chakra also energizes the legs to a substantial degree. It is clairvoyantly observed that when a man is urinating, his sex chakra and meng mein chakra produce more orange prana, which is used in expelling and eliminating waste matter from the body. The sex chakra is the lower or physical creative center.

The *meng mein chakra* has eight petals and contains orange, yellow and orange-red pranas. The meng mein chakra controls and energizes the kidneys, adrenal glands, and to a certain extent, other internal organs. It acts as a pumping station for the red pranic energy from the basic chakra and is responsible for the upward flow of pranic energy in the spine. Please note that we have indicated in the treatment sections that this chakra should be used with caution.

The *navel chakra* has eight petals and predominantly contains yellow, green, blue, red and violet pranas. It also contains a little orange prana. This chakra controls and energizes the small intestine, the lower large intestine, and the appendix. The navel chakra produces the "synthetic ki" which facilitates or helps in the circulation of prana within the meridians. "Synthetic ki" facilitates the drawing in of prana by the etheric body. Persons with more "synthetic ki" can draw in more prana than those with less "synthetic ki." People with less "synthetic ki" feel low during poor weather.

The *spleen chakra* has six petals and contains red, orange, yellow, green, blue, and violet pranas. The spleen chakra draws in a lot of air prana and energizes other major chakras by distributing the digested pranas to them. In other words, the spleen chakra energizes the entire bioplasmic body, thereby energizing the visible physical body.

The spleen chakra is closely related to the navel chakra. When the navel chakra is energized or activated, the spleen chakra becomes energized or activated, drawing in more air prana and increasing the pranic energy level of the entire body.

A person can be energized just by concentrating on the navel chakra. By concentrating on the navel chakra, it becomes activated and energized. This in turn activates and energizes the spleen chakra which energizes the other chakras; thereby energizing the entire body.

The *solar plexus chakra* has ten petals and contains red, orange, yellow, green and blue pranas. It also contains a little violet prana. This chakra controls and energizes the liver, pancreas, stomach, large intestine, diaphragm and to a certain degree energizes the adrenal glands, the small intestine, the heart, the lungs and other parts of the body. It is easier to energize the pancreas through the back solar plexus chakra. An exhausted person can be revitalized rapidly by energizing the solar plexus chakra.

The solar plexus chakra is one of the most important chakras because it controls and energizes so many vital organs. It is easily disturbed or imbalanced by negative emotions. The solar plexus chakra is the center of lower emotions.

When a person is very angry, the solar plexus chakra pulsates erratically. This causes the diaphragm to move erratically, resulting in irregular shallow breathing.

When a person has a bowel movement, the solar plexus chakra, the navel chakra and the basic chakra produce a lot of orange and yellow pranas. When yellow prana comes in contact with orange prana, a triggering effect on the large intestine is produced. This is the reason why orange or yellow prana or both are used in treating constipation.

The *heart chakra* has twelve petals. The front heart chakra contains a lot of golden prana with some red prana. It controls and energizes the heart and the thymus gland. The back heart chakra contains orange and red pranas with some golden and yellow pranas. It controls and energizes primarily the lungs, and to a certain degree, the heart. The heart chakra is the center of higher or refined emotions. It is very closely related to the solar plexus chakra since both are emotional centers. To agitate the solar plexus chakra is also to agitate the heart chakra. This is why negative emotions have detrimental effects on the heart in the long run.

The *throat chakra* has sixteen petals and predominantly contains blue prana with some green and violet pranas. A lot of green prana is produced when a person is eating. It controls and energizes the throat, the thyroid glands, the parathyroid glands and the lymphatic system. Malfunctioning of this chakra manifests as throat related ailments, such as goiter, sore throat, loss of voice, and asthma. The throat chakra is the center of the lower or concrete mind or lower mental faculty and it is also the higher creative center.

The *ajna chakra* has ninety-six petals and is divided into two divisions. Each division has forty-eight petals. With some people, one of the divisions is predominantly light yellow, and the other division is predominantly light violet. Others have whitish-green in one of the divisions, and light violet on the other. The predominating color pranas in the ajna is not the same in all people. The color of the ajna chakra also changes with the psychological state. The ajna chakra is the center of the higher or abstract mind and it is also the will or directive center. It controls and energizes the pituitary gland and the entire body. The ajna chakra is called the master chakra because it controls all the major chakras, the endocrine glands and the vital organs. Malfunctioning of this chakra manifests as diseases related to the endocrine glands and the eyes.

The *forehead chakra* has 144 petals divided into twelve divisions. Each division contains twelve petals. This chakra controls and energizes the pineal gland and the nervous system. Malfunctioning of the forehead chakra may manifest as loss of memory, paralysis and epilepsy. The forehead chakra contains violet, blue, red, orange, yellow and green pranas. The forehead chakra is the center of the lower Buddhic or cosmic consciousness.

The *crown chakra* has 960 external petals and twelve inner petals. The crown chakra is the only chakra with two sets of petals. It can also be considered to have an inner and outer chakra. The inner chakra looks like the front heart chakra. The twelve inner petals contain predominantly golden prana and the 960 external petals contain violet, blue, green-yellow and orange-red pranas. The crown chakra controls and energizes the brain and the pineal gland. Malfunctioning of this chakra may manifest as disease related to the pineal gland and brain, which may also manifest as physical or psychological illnesses.

The crown chakra is the center of the higher Buddhic or cosmic consciousness. The mental faculty can be compared to a blind man while the Buddhic consciousness to a person who can see. For a blind man to have an idea of the shape of an elephant, he has to spend a considerable amount of time touching the elephant and trying to deduce and synthesize the data gathered, while a person who can see will be able to immediately know the shape of an elephant. Buddhic consciousness is understanding a subject matter not through a long period of study nor through inductive or deductive reasoning, but through immediate "direct comprehension or perception." Another term for Buddhic consciousness is Christ consciousness. Through Buddhic consciousness one feels oneness with all, oneness with God. It is through Christ consciousness that one feels loving-kindness to all.

ENERGIZING WITH COLOR PRANAS

There are three methods of energizing with color pranas—by visualizing, using the chakral technique, or combining visualization and chakral techniques.

In the visualization approach, you simply do pranic breathing and visualize the specific color prana coming out of your hand. Do not visualize the specific color prana being drawn in; just visualize the specific color prana projecting out of your hand chakra. For example, if you want to energize with green prana, you just simply visualize green light projecting out of your hand chakra. Practice regularly so you can be sure that the color prana projected is the expected one. It is quite possible that you may be visualizing green or blue prana projecting out of your hand chakra but what is actually coming out is light red prana. Or you may be trying to project light red prana but what is coming out is dark red. Practice is necessary to become proficient in projecting color pranas.

In the chakral technique, you simply choose a source chakra that provides the specific color prana or pranas required. For example, if you want to treat an infection with blue or green-blue prana, you can draw in prana from your throat chakra and project the blue or green-blue prana through your hand chakra. This can simply be done by doing pranic breathing and simultaneously concentrating on your throat chakra and your hand chakra. You should form an intention to draw in prana from your throat chakra and project it out through the hand chakra. This is the same as the energizing technique taught in elementary pranic healing. Instead of concentrating on the left and right hand chakras, you just simply concentrate on your throat chakra and your hand chakra. Similarly, if you want to treat a fresh wound using orange-red prana, you can use the basic chakra as the source chakra and project it out through your hand chakra.

Sometimes, just using the chakral technique is not enough to produce the right type and shade of color prana. It is necessary to combine the visualization technique with the chakral technique. For example, if you want to strengthen an internal organ with light red prana, concentrate on the basic chakra and visualize light red prana projecting out of your hand chakra. If you just concentrate on the basic chakra without visualizing your hand projecting light red prana, you might be projecting orange-red instead of red prana. Red prana is strengthening. But most internal organs cannot withstand too much orange prana or orange-red prana because they will be physically damaged.

You can perform an experiment by transforming white prana to color prana by an act of will. This experiment requires the help of a clairvoyant or a person with auric sight. Get a glass of water and place it in front of you. Draw in vitality globules or white prana from the surroundings into the water by willing and visualizing the globules gathering and forming into a white ball of light. Bring the ball of white prana (white ball of light) down into the water. Visualize and transform the white ball of light into the specific color prana that you want. Get feedback from the clairvoyant whether you have been successful in drawing in a substantial amount of prana into the water, and whether the white prana has been transformed into the desired color prana. Let the clairvoyant observe the energized water for several hours and for several days to see whether the white prana has been permanently transformed into the desired color prana.

At first, you may encounter problems in gathering the vitality globules and transforming them into the specific color prana. The transformed prana may not be so steady. For example, you may visualize green prana and get other color pranas instead. Not all of the vitality globules are transformed into the expected color prana. The transformed color prana is not stable and the color vacillates between green and white. If the green prana is still quite unstable, more "willing" or visualization has to be done. These problems can be overcome by lots of practice.

Some healers use their eyes to energize patients. This practice, when done frequently for a long period of time or for even a short period of time, will damage the eyes. When you energize, an etheric or bioplasmic link is established between the projecting chakra and the diseased part. Diseased etheric matter or diseased bioplasmic matter may sometimes be absorbed by the projecting chakra through the etheric link. That is why the eyes will be damaged if used regularly to project prana to the diseased parts. Sometimes healers experience diseased bioplasmic matter creeping up to their arms when they are energizing with their hand chakras.

It is not advisable to regularly energize directly from your major chakra to the diseased part of the patient for the same reason. It is better to energize with the hand chakra or finger chakra since the hands and fingers are easier to clean and are not too delicate compared to the eyes, brain or heart.

Sometimes, even though the healer is using his or her hand chakra to energize the affected part, he or she also unconsciously energizes with the eyes, thereby damaging the eyes in the long run. This usually happens to the healer who tends to stare intensely at the affected part when healing another person.

Advanced General Sweeping

In general sweeping, use first light green prana to clean, decongest and disinfect the patient, then light red prana to strengthen the entire body. It is best to go through the following procedures:

1) Visualize a brilliant ball of light above the crown chakra.

2) Apply a downward sweeping movement and visualize light whitish-green prana coming down from the ball, filling and cleansing the entire

body, with more emphasis on the front part of the body. Visualize all the front major chakras as clean and bright.

3) Apply another downward sweeping movement and visualize light whitish-green prana cleansing the entire body with emphasis on the back part of the body. Visualize the spine and all the back major chakras as clean and bright.

4) Apply another downward sweeping movement and visualize light whitish-green prana cleansing the entire body with emphasis on the important internal organs. Visualize the internal organs as bright light red.

5) Apply another downward sweeping movement two times and visualize light whitish-red prana energizing and strengthening all the important internal organs. Visualize all the health rays as straight and bright, especially on the affected area.

6) Apply another downward sweeping movement and visualize light whitish-red prana energizing and strengthening the bones and the muscles. Visualize all the health rays as straight and bright. You may repeat the entire process several times.

This advanced form of general sweeping cleanses, energizes and strengthens the entire body. It can relieve asthma and can be used to treat chill and fever. It can be very beneficial to patients who have just undergone surgery and should be used before and after surgery. However, this technique cannot be used on any patient who has or has had a sexually transmittable disease such as AIDS, herpes, gonorrhea, syphilis, etc.

Advanced Localized Sweeping

Visualize light whitish-green prana surrounding your hand about six inches in diameter and about one to one-and-a-half feet long. Apply localized sweeping on the affected part and simultaneously visualize the diseased grayish matter being removed and the affected part being filled with prana. This advanced localized sweeping is quite effective and can remove mild toothaches, headaches and other minor ailments with just one or two sweeping movements.

Decongesting or Loosening

If the diseased bioplasmic matter is difficult to remove, or is quite stubborn, it would be advisable to energize first with light whitish-green prana for two breathing cycles, followed by light whitish-orange prana for two breathing cycles to loosen the stubborn diseased bioplasmic matter. Please note the sequence, green prana before orange prana. This approach is much safer. The removal of the loosened diseased bioplasmic matter can be facilitated by projecting light whitish-yellow prana when applying localized sweeping. If cleansing is done properly, partial relief or improvement should occur. For delicate organs like the brain, eyes, and heart, it is not advisable to use orange prana.

Cleansing Delicate Organs

Sometimes an ailment can be caused by partial clogging of very fine bioplasmic channels. An example would be nearsightedness or farsightedness. Used-up prana and diseased bioplasmic matter in the eyes can be loosened and broken down into very fine particles by energizing with light whitish-green prana. Project light whitish-yellow prana to group together these fine particles for easier removal and apply localized sweeping. Light yellow prana is preferable to blue prana because blue prana tends to remove not only the used-up prana but also the fresh prana. Please note that light green prana is used in loosening and cleansing delicate organs like the eyes and the brain. Orange prana is not used because it is too powerful and may result in undesirable side effects. There is no point in taking unnecessary risks.

Energizing Time

There is no definite time allowed for energizing. It is left to the healer's discretion. Certain factors have to be considered, such as the condition of the patient, the severity of the ailment, the rate of pranic energy consumption of the affected part, and the proficiency of the healer. Some healers prefer to energize intensely and rapidly while others prefer to energize moderately and gradually. Advanced healers can energize a chakra in just a few seconds. Color prana is projected for only three or four seconds. For mild ailments, the entire treatment may take less than a minute.

For ordinary infections, energizing with blue prana and green prana for five to seven breathing cycles would be sufficient. For very severe types of infection, energizing would require ten to fifteen minutes once every two hours for the next eight hours. These are just rough guidelines. You will have to use your own discretion. It is very important to rescan and determine whether the energizing is sufficient or not.

Frequency of Treatment

In emergency cases, treatments should be given at faster intervals until the condition stabilizes. For severe ailments, treatments should be given once a day or once every two days. For less severe types of ailments, it may be given once a week. Ordinary ailments usually require only one or two healing sessions. It is important that the rate of healing be much faster than the rate of deterioration. That is why emergency or severe cases should be treated at more frequent intervals.

Treating Infants and Old People

In treating infants, it is advisable to avoid using dark green prana because it may affect the future development of the organs being energized. Using localized sweeping and energizing with white prana would be sufficient to clean and energize the infant. There is no point in taking unnecessary risk, no matter how minimal it is.

In treating both infants and older people, it is advisable to avoid using dark blue prana, especially in the solar plexus and heart chakras, because of its strong inhibiting effects on the functioning of the organs.

Invocation Before Healing

It is better to invoke the aid of Divine Providence before healing the patient to make the pranic treatment easier, more effective and safer. If the patient is suffering from severe ailments then request the Lord to assign a healing angel to remain with the patient after the treatment to hasten the healing process. We discussed this earlier.

Infection and Inflammation

For treating infection and inflammation, use light whitish-green prana, then light whitish-blue prana. Blue prana is for disinfecting, inhibiting, containing, localizing, cooling and soothing effects. Green prana has disinfecting, decongesting and cleansing effects. Green prana breaks down dirty diseased bioplasmic matter. For severe types of infection, use violet prana because it has the strongest disinfecting effect. Other pranas also have disinfecting properties but of lesser effectivity.

Blue prana disinfects by its inhibiting action, its localizing and containing effects, and also by stimulating the production of antibodies. Green prana acts by breaking down the diseased germs—either directly or indirectly—by stimulating the production of antibodies or substances with breaking down effects on the germs. When greenish-blue (approximately 30% greenish prana and 70% blue prana) is used, the potency is increased several times. Preferably, greenish-blue prana should not be used in general sweeping because some patients cannot withstand it and it may bring forth severe detrimental effects.

Greenish-blue prana is used for severe infection or inflammation and should be used with caution on delicate organs. It is also used to treat food poisoning and insect bites on the arms and legs. It should preferably not be used on people under twenty or over forty-five because it has a constrictive effect on delicate organs. When used regularly for a certain period of time, it may have damaging effects.

Strengthening

Light whitish-red prana is used to strengthen organs or parts that have been weakened. Energize the affected part with light whitish-green prana for two breathing cycles, then with light whitish-red prana for seven breathing cycles. In cases where the parts or organs to be treated are inflamed, energize first with light whitish-green prana for two breathing cycles, then with light whitish-blue prana for seven breathing cycles, and finally with light whitish-red prana for two breathing cycles to strengthen the inflamed parts or organs. Light whitish-red prana is safer to use than light red prana. Avoid using dark red prana as this may cause further inflammation.

Inhibiting

Blue prana can be used to inhibit a chakra and its corresponding organs. For example, the overproduction of gastric juices can be inhibited by first cleansing the solar plexus chakra with white prana and second, by energizing it with blue prana. It is clairvoyantly observed that patients recovering from gastric ulcers have a lot of blue prana in the solar plexus chakra.

Disintegrating Deposits

Green prana and orange prana are used in disintegrating deposits. Clean the affected area and energize with green prana then energize with orange prana to dissolve and eliminate the deposits. Blue prana is used first to localize the disintegrating effect of the pranic energy on the affected part.

Acute Allergy

All types of prana can relieve allergies, but the best type of prana for allergies is red prana. There are certain types of acute or severe allergies that can be relieved only by using red prana. There is a severe skin allergy that looks like severe skin infection but does not respond to any antibiotic treatment. This type of allergy can be healed by energizing the affected part with red prana or by wrapping a red cloth near the affected area. Energize the affected part with light green prana for one breathing cycle, then with light red prana for five to eight breathing cycles.

To cure the patient of allergy and not just relieve it, cleanse the ajna chakra and the basic chakra. Energize the basic chakra with red prana for seven breathing cycles and the ajna chakra with light whitish-violet prana for four breathing cycles. The bones in the arms and legs have to be energized with light red prana. This is done by energizing the arms through the hand chakras and the armpit chakras with light red prana for four breathing cycles for each chakra. Energize the legs through the sole chakras and the hip chakras with light red prana for four breathing cycles for each chakra. Visualize light red prana going inside the bones. Repeat the treatment twice a week for the first few weeks then reduce it to once a week. Partial malfunctioning of the liver or the kidney may also cause the allergy. In such cases, also treat the solar plexus chakra and the liver or the meng mein chakra and kidneys.

188 • PRANIC HEALING

HOW TO ACTIVATE THE CHAKRA

Activating your chakra or that of the patient's is needed for more advanced and faster healing. A simple method of activating the chakra would be to visualize and will the chakra to increase in size and brightness while simultaneously energizing it with red prana (for solar plexus and downward), or white-violet prana (for heart chakra and upwards). Visualize the chakra as increasing from three to five inches. It should be visualized as dazzling. The key factor is in willing. Do this for five breathing cycles.

Master Healing Technique

Activating and energizing the basic and meng mein chakras is a very important technique in healing. The basic chakra energizes the entire physical body. Activating and energizing the basic chakra alone would increase the pranic energy level of the body to a limited degree. As stated earlier, the meng mein chakra acts as a sort of pump to facilitate the distribution of red pranic energy from the basic chakra to the other parts of the body. To be more accurate, it acts as an accelerator, since it increases the rate of vibration of the prana coming from the basic chakra. So the rate of vibration of pranic energy from the basic chakra is higher when it comes out of the meng mein chakra than before going into it. Without activating and energizing the meng mein chakra, the pranic energy from the basic chakra would have difficulty spreading rapidly to other parts of the body. This is like having a big factory in full production with a very poor marketing department to distribute the product.

When these two chakras are activated and energized, pranic energy from the basic chakra will gush out with tremendous speed through the back bioplasmic channel (or meridian) and spread to all parts of the body. The entire body and the internal organs are energized and strengthened and become much brighter and more reddish. Activating and energizing the basic and meng mein chakras is considered a master healing technique. This healing technique can be used to treat many types of ailments.

This master healing technique can be used for energizing and strengthening the internal organs and the entire body. This technique is very useful for patients who are weak or very depleted and have ailments involving the internal organs. With some depleted patients, the energizing and strengthening effects are almost instantaneous. It can also be used to make strong young athletes even stronger.

The master healing technique can be used to greatly increase and strengthen the body's defense mechanism. This technique is used on severe types of infection. It means that if your patient has a severe eye or lung infection, then this healing technique can be used. Do not use this healing technique on patients with venereal disease or who have a history of venereal disease, since this technique produces a lot of red prana which will activate the venereal germs, and thus worsen the condition of the patient.

This master healing technique accelerates the healing process several times and can be used on some severe types of ailments. Exceptions are when the patient has high blood pressure or is suffering from pranic congestion throughout the body, which can sometimes happen to esoteric students who overpractice or incorrectly practice advanced types of yoga.

This technique can be used on emergency cases. Unconscious patients who are on the verge of dying can be revived by using this technique. When the basic and the meng mein chakra are energized, red pranic energy from the basic chakra rushes up to energize the brain and the entire body. This technique also accelerates tissue repair (or the growth rate of cells) and can be used on patients before and after surgery.

The master healing technique can also be used as a supplemental or supportive healing technique together with the main pranic treatment. For example, if the patient has a lung ailment, then the lungs should be treated (main pranic treatment) and the basic and the meng mein chakras should be activated and energized to further increase the rate of healing. The main pranic treatment can be given before or after activating and energizing the basic and the meng mein chakras.

One of the effects of using this powerful technique is that it tends to increase the sexual drive. Patients should be advised about this and be told to avoid sexual activity to prevent pranic depletion and to accelerate the healing process.

Work with the technique as follows:

1) Apply localized sweeping to the basic and meng mein chakras. With some patients, it is necessary to clean both the back and front channels or apply general sweeping several times.

2) Activate and energize the basic and meng mein chakras for five to seven breathing cycles. Visualize the basic chakra increasing in size up to five inches in diameter and the meng mein chakra up to three to four inches

in diameter. Making the meng mein over four inches will result in hypertension.

For advanced healers, the will power should not be used in full force. Otherwise, the patient may suffer undesirable side effects due to overactivating the basic and meng mein chakras. Rescan the basic and meng mein chakras frontally and sideways to determine the degree of activation.

This powerful healing technique is quite safe as long as the following guidelines are observed:

1) Never use this powerful healing technique on pregnant women. The energy generated can overwhelm or destroy the delicate chakras of the unborn baby. There is the possibility of miscarriage or the baby may be stillborn.

2) Do not activate and energize more than seven cycles. For powerful healers, the number of breathing cycles has to be reduced. The patient may be overenergized resulting in high blood pressure and possible allergy throughout the body. He or she may feel quite weak and uneasy for the next few days because of too much pranic energy. Also, the brain will be affected and the patient may find it difficult to concentrate.

3) Do not energize the spleen chakra if the basic and meng mein chakras have been activated and energized or will be activated and energized. This will cause the body to be overenergized. The side effects will be similar to overactivating and overenergizing the basic and meng mein chakras, except that they may be even more severe. This is similar to a blown fuse or melted wire due to too much electric current. Do not activate or energize the navel chakra if the basic and meng mein chakras have been or will be activated. By activating or energizing the navel chakra, the spleen chakra becomes partially activated or energized.

4) This technique should not be used on patients with high blood pressure and on patients suffering from glaucoma.

5) It should not be used on patients suffering from leprosy because it would only worsen the ailment.

6) It should not be used on patients suffering from cancer. This master healing technique tends to increase the growth rate of cells, therefore it will greatly increase the growth rate of the cancer cells, thereby worsening the condition. It should also not be applied on patients with cirrhosis of

the liver, or any inflammation of the liver, because it would only worsen the condition.

7) Do not use this healing technique on leukemia patients since it tends to increase the white blood cells, thereby worsening the condition.

8) Do not use this healing technique on patients suffering from severe heart ailments. The heart has a strong tendency to draw or attract pranic energy. The use of this advanced healing technique on a patient with a serious heart ailment may result in pranic congestion manifesting as cardiac arrest.

9) This healing technique should be used only on those patients whose ages range from fifteen to forty-five. Infants and children may suffer brain damage due to too much pranic energy rushing upward. With children, their chakras are not quite developed and to subject them to intense pranic energy may cause serious imbalance in the bioplasmic body. For older patients, this technique will have detrimental effects since their bodies and endocrine glands have atrophied and cannot withstand too much pranic energy. As discussed in earlier chapters, infants, children, weak and old patients should be gently and gradually energized!

This master healing technique can be toned down by just energizing the basic and meng mein chakras without substantially activating them. This means that you do not visualize or will the chakra to become bigger and brighter; you simply energize it. Energizing without activating the basic and meng mein chakras can be used for patients whose age ranges from twelve to sixty. It should not be used on infants. This milder form of master healing technique is still quite potent and can easily energize and strengthen a depleted patient in a short time. The same guidelines should be followed when using the milder form of master healing technique.

The master healing technique should only be used by experienced healers, not by beginners.

HOW TO ACTIVATE THE ADRENAL GLANDS

The adrenal glands can be activated to temporarily increase physical strength and stamina.

1) Apply the master healing technique.

2) Will or direct pranic energy to go to the adrenal glands.

3) Activate the back solar plexus chakra for five to seven cycles.

4) Will or direct pranic energy to go to the adrenal glands.

5) After the required physical feat has been done, normalize the meng mein chakra, the basic chakra, and the back solar plexus chakra.

6) The same guidelines used in the master healing technique should be followed. Please read the guidelines thoroughly before applying this technique. This technique can also be used to treat emergency ailments or cases.

ACTIVATING AND ENERGIZING THE BASIC CHAKRA AND THE PERINEUM CHAKRA

To facilitate the flow of pranic energy from the basic chakra to the legs in order to strengthen them, just activate and energize the basic chakra and the perineum minor chakra. The act of activating and energizing the perineum minor chakra is like turning on a water faucet. You do not have to ask your patient to assume an embarrassing position just to activate and energize the perineum minor chakra. Just visualize the perineum in front of your hand chakra, then proceed to activate and energize it. Five to seven breathing cycles would be sufficient to activate and energize the basic chakra and the perineum minor chakra.

INSTANTANEOUS HEALING OF A FRESH WOUND

Instantaneous healing of a wound is applicable only if the wound is fresh. The rate of instantaneous healing ranges from twenty minutes to one or two hours. How long it will take depends on the patient's body, the proficiency of the healer, and the size of the wound. The healer may take several short rests when energizing.

The basic chakra, which is the source of orange-red prana, is used in instantaneous healing of a wound. The red prana is about sixty percent and the orange prana as about forty percent. The red and orange pranas are projected simultaneously and not one after the other. The effect is quite different if orange prana is projected first, then red prana or vice versa compared to orange-red prana. Orange prana has a cleansing or expelling effect which may increase the bleeding. Red prana has a strengthening effect, and to a certain degree increases the growth rate of cells. Orange-red prana accelerates the growth rate of cells, thereby causing rapid, if not instantaneous, healing of the fresh wound.

It is important that the basic chakra of both the patient and the healer should be activated and energized. This is necessary in order to have enough pranic energy to produce instantaneous healing of the wound. To use the basic chakra of the healer alone is not enough. It would take a longer time before the wound will be fully or substantially healed. The instantaneous healing technique, the master healing technique, and some advanced healing techniques were taught me by my respected teacher, Mei Ling.

The procedure is as follows:

1) Activate and energize the patient's basic chakra for five to seven breathing cycles, then activate and energize your basic chakra for five to seven breathing cycles. Or you may activate and energize simultaneously both your basic chakra and the patient's basic chakra. This is done by activating and energizing your patient's basic chakra and simultaneously concentrating and activating your basic chakra. Visualize your basic chakra and the patient's basic chakra as becoming bigger and brighter for five to seven breathing cycles.

2) Energize the fresh wound with pranic energy from your basic chakra and the patient's basic chakra. This can be done by applying short circuiting on the patient's basic chakra and on the wound. Short circuiting is done by drawing pranic energy from the patient's basic chakra with one of your hand chakras, then directing it to the wound with your other hand chakra. Put one of your hands near the patient's basic chakra and the other near the wound. Concentrate simultaneously on your basic chakra and hand chakras. Visualize the wound being energized with orange-red prana, and as healing and closing. You do not have to visualize your basic chakra and the patient's basic chakra. This is unnecessary and would only make you tense and tired. Just visualize the orange-red prana coming out of your hand chakra but be sure to concentrate on your basic chakra and on the other hand chakra simultaneously. Your visualization does not have to be clear. What is important is the intention or the willing. Continue with

the treatment until the wound is completely healed. You may take several short rests when treating.

3) Instead of using the short-circuiting technique to draw in pranic energy from the patient's basic chakra, you can just simply will the pranic energy from his or her basic chakra to go to the wound. It would be advantageous if your meng mein chakra and the patient's meng mein chakra are activated and energized to facilitate the flow of pranic energy. By activating your meng mein chakra and the patient's meng mein chakra, the healing rate of the wound is further increased. If the cut is on the leg, then the patient's perineum minor chakra should be activated and energized. The instructions may seem long and complicated but it is actually quite simple and short.

Your initial reaction to this teaching could, of course, be of doubt. This is quite normal, even for students of esoteric science. Does instantaneous healing of a wound require an exceptional person? No, but the healer should at least be proficient in intermediate pranic healing. Try it several times and judge for yourself. The first few sessions may take you longer to heal and the wound may not be one hundred percent healed, but with practice you can become very proficient at it. If you want to become a good healer, just reading and speculating about pranic healing is not enough. The only way to learn pranic healing is through lots and lots of practice and experiments.

This instantaneous healing of a wound technique is used on fresh wounds. It cannot be used on delicate internal organs because too much orange prana may cause damage to the internal organ being treated.

Orange-red prana is not used in healing the brain and the nervous system. Using it would result in the production of abnormal or mongoloid cells which would only result in more harm.

It is advisable that you experiment with small wounds first, then gradually go to bigger ones. With a small wound, you must first energize it to stop the bleeding. You may use blue prana, white prana or orange-red prana to stop the bleeding. Clean the wound and remove the blood by using cotton and alcohol. Energize the wound for twenty minutes and observe the result. Continue energizing if the wound is not sufficiently or completely healed. With bigger or surgical wounds, the procedure is more or less the same. It is important to stop the bleeding first, then clean and remove the blood before stitching or taping the wound together. It is then energized for instantaneous healing. I have experimented with instantaneous healing of small wounds and have obtained very good results.

This technique can probably be used on a patient whose finger has been accidentally cut-off. You will of course need the help of a surgeon to re-attach the finger. The patient should immediately contact the emergency room at his or her local hospital for surgery. In this case, pranic healing would be used as an adjunct to surgical treatment.

You may use pranic invocative healing to obtain the help of mighty angels or *mahadevas* to accelerate further the healing of the wound.

BROKEN BONES

Light orange-yellow prana (60 percent yellow, 40 percent orange) is used for rapid healing of fractured bones. You can use the basic chakra as the source for orange-yellow prana. Visualize the projected prana as orange-yellow and energize for ten to fifteen minutes. Energize the affected part with light orange-red prana for five breathing cycles.

RAPID HEALING OF OLD WOUNDS AND BURNS

Green prana is not used on fresh wounds because it is slower in effect and tends to make the wound wet or watery. It can be used in the rapid healing of old wounds and burns. A lot of green prana is required for breaking down dead cells. To heal old wounds and burns, energize the affected part with greenish-red prana (40 percent greenish prana and 60 percent red prana) for fifteen minutes. You may use the solar plexus chakra or the navel chakra as a source chakra for green-red prana. Repeat the treatment once or twice a day.

The healing of old wounds may take several days or longer, depending upon the age and the condition of the patient's body, the size of the wound, and the proficiency of the healer. A big wound has a much higher rate of pranic energy consumption than a small wound, therefore a small wound would heal at a faster rate. A vegetarian whose bioplasmic body or etheric body is much brighter, denser and healthier would generally heal at a much faster rate than those who are not vegetarian. Some small old wounds can be completely healed in a few hours by continuously energizing it with greenish-red prana alternated with orange-red prana.

For fresh burns, cleanse immediately and energize alternately with green prana and blue prana, until the patient is completely relieved. Do not use red or orange prana, since it will produce blisters.

REGENERATION

Greenish-violet prana (40 percent greenish prana and 60 percent violet prana) and greenish-yellow prana (40 percent greenish prana and 60 percent yellow prana) are used to regenerate damaged brain, nerve cells and internal organs. Light whitish-red prana is used to strengthen the organ being treated with the above color pranas. The rate of healing depends on the degree of damage, the physical condition of the patient, the karmic factor, and the healer's degree of proficiency. It may take several days, weeks, months, or an indefinite period of time.

Clean the affected chakra and organ with light whitish-green prana. Energize with light whitish-greenish violet prana, then energize with light whitish-greenish yellow prana. Energize the affected organ with light whitish-red prana to strengthen it. Repeat the treatment twice a week. You may use the crown chakra as the source chakra for greenish-violet prana, violet prana and greenish-yellow prana.

Practitioners will need to determine the amount of time needed for cleansing and energizing and adjust as necessary for each patient.

MORE ABOUT KARMA

When a person does something with intention whether positively or negatively, the karmic effect is tenfold. This is the principle behind tithing. When you plant a grain of rice, you harvest not only a grain of rice but you harvest many times what you have planted. When you plant a mango seed, you get a mango tree that would produce many mango fruits.

When spiritual aspirants, including pranic healers, do something with intention—whether positively or negatively—the karmic effect is one-hundred-fold. This is no exaggeration but is to be taken literally. To deliberately misuse one's power or what has been taught in this book would have a devastating or crushing effect on oneself. It is wiser and better to do good deeds rather than negative deeds.

You do not have to blindly accept my words. You can experiment by doing something not too negative and observe what happens. You can also try doing something positive, like tithing, and observe what happens. Very often the karmic effect is not on a lump sum basis but is done on a piecemeal or staggered basis, but still the negative karmic effects are devastating. I have personally experimented and experienced the immediate effects of both positive and negative karma.

The law of karma is not fatalistic, but is self-determining or self-directing. It is self-determining in the sense that karmic effects originate from yourself; therefore, you can deliberately produce positive or negative karmic effects by setting in motion positive or negative causal factors. It also means that you are responsible and accountable for your deeds, words, and feelings/thoughts. You cannot blame other people, your parents, your environment or some unseen forces for your problems or troubles. If you get in trouble, then you should get out of it with or without outside help. If you are experiencing a lot of bad luck, or your condition is restrictive, or you are subjected to injustices, then meditate and learn whatever lessons are to be learned from them. Do good deeds to generate good karma. Definitely work hard and intelligently to improve your conditions. By learning your lessons, by doing good deeds, and by working hard and intelligently, you can reverse an adverse condition. It is by working out or overcoming negative karma that one is purified and gains inner strength and wisdom.

ORANGE-YELLOW PRANA

Orange-yellow prana is not used to heal fresh or old wounds because its use tends to form ugly scars or keloids. Orange-yellow prana is used for skin or bone grafting. It is projected on the area where the bone or skin was taken. This is done for twenty to thirty minutes per healing session. Orange-red prana is less effective in such a case because it does not have the ability to "fill" the hole or gap where the skin or bone was taken. Use the basic chakra as the source chakra for orange-yellow prana.

To stabilize and prevent possible infection on the grafted bone or skin, energize it with light green prana for five breathing cycles and then with light blue prana for five breathing cycles. To strengthen and facilitate the assimilation of the grafted bone or skin, energize with light whitish-red prana for four breathing cycles and then with light whitish-yellow prana for four breathing cycles.

PRANIC HEALING APPLIED IN SURGERY

Pranic healing is also useful for treating patients before, during and after surgery. Pranic healing can be used to reduce bleeding, to minimize the possibility of infection, to strengthen the body, the part or organ to be operated on, and to accelerate the rate of recovery.

Several days before surgery, the body can be strengthened by applying general sweeping and by activating and energizing the basic and the meng mein chakras. The area and organs to be operated on and the nearby chakras should also be cleansed and energized several times. Just before surgery, the part or organ to be operated on should be energized with light whitish-green prana for two breathing cycles, with light whitish-blue prana for eight breathing cycles to reduce bleeding and to prevent possible infection; and then with light whitish-red prana for two breathing cycles to strengthen the area to be operated on. The major chakras nearest the part to be operated on should also be energized with white prana.

During surgery, if required, the healer may apply pranic healing to reduce bleeding, and to clean, energize, and strengthen the entire body, a specific organ, or a specific major chakra (or chakras).

After the surgery, general sweeping should be applied several times a day to clean the entire body. The etheric body or the bioplasmic body is grayish after the operation. Chakras that are depleted have to be cleansed and energized. The area operated on should be energized with light green prana for two breathing cycles, with light blue prana for seven breathing cycles, and with light orange-red prana to accelerate the healing of the wound. The treatment should be continued for the next several days or weeks.

RAPID GROWTH

When red and yellow prana are used one after the other, a rapid growth of cells is produced. This combination of prana can be used to stimulate hair growth. This is done by applying localized sweeping to the head area, then energizing it with a little light blue prana in order to localize the prana that will be applied later. Energize the affected part with light whitish-red prana, then with light whitish-yellow prana. Repeat the treatment for at least twice a week for as long as necessary. Never use dark red prana and dark yellow prana. Also never energize with yellow-red prana or red prana and yellow prana simultaneously because it will produce disruptive, if not destructive, effects on the patient.

This can also be applied to plants to produce faster growth. You may perform an experiment for about one month on the rapid growth of plants with the use of red prana and yellow prana. When energizing the plant, project the red prana first, followed by yellow prana; never energize with both pranas simultaneously. Visualize the pranic energy going into the root and into the core of the plant. Yellow-red prana is very powerful and would result in too rapid a multiplication of cells, resulting in the destruction of the plant or tree being energized. This prana is never used in healing.

Red prana, and yellow prana, can also be used to facilitate the assimilation and acceptance by the body of a newly transplanted organ. This would reduce the risk of rejection.

INCREASING RESISTANCE AGAINST INFECTION

Activating and energizing the meng mein chakra and the basic chakra is used to increase the body's resistance against infection. For more information, see the Master Healing Technique on page 188. A safer technique, however, would be to energize the navel chakra, the palms and the soles with light violet prana.

TO STOP BLEEDING

Different types of prana can be used to stop the bleeding in most cases. To heal a wound that will not stop bleeding, or one that takes a long time for the blood to clot, energize the wound with blue prana for four breathing cycles or until the bleeding stops. Energize the wound with orange-red prana to facilitate the healing process.

For nose bleeding, energize with white prana or light blue prana for four breathing cycles or until the bleeding stops.

For hemophilia, energize with greenish-blue prana until the bleeding stops. Not blue prana, then green prana, but both pranas simultaneously. This technique is based on the instruction given to me by my teacher, Mei Ling.

Greenish-blue prana is not used in general sweeping because some patients may experience adverse reaction or side effects.

STEPS IN HEALING

1) Interview and observe the patient carefully.

2) Scan all the major chakras, the relevant minor chakras, the important organs and the spine thoroughly. An affected chakra which seems unrelated to the ailment and is quite far from the location of the ailment may be a major contributing factor to the ailment. Thorough scanning is the key to proper treatment.

3) Clean and energize the chakras and organs to be treated. Use the necessary color pranas to correct or remedy the ailment. In cases where you are not sure of what color pranas to use, work with white prana. For instance, a patient with a lung infection should be treated with green prana, then with blue prana to disinfect, then with light orange prana to expel diseased bioplasmic matter, toxins and germs in the lungs, then with light red prana to strengthen the lungs. White prana may be used at the end or during the treatment to dilute the potency of the color prana used and to harmonize the condition.

4) For pranic congestion, cleansing should be emphasized. For pranic depletion, energizing should be emphasized. The projected prana should be stabilized! Be sure to rescan the treated parts.

5) The treatment can be divided into two parts—relieving the patient and correcting the conditions causing the ailment.

For example, the healer may relieve a patient of a headache by treating the head area and correcting the condition by treating the eyes if the cause of the headache is due to eyestrain. The healer can also relieve an asthmatic patient by treating the throat chakra, the secondary throat chakra, and the back heart chakra. This condition can be corrected by treating the ajna chakra, the basic chakra and the bones.

There are cases in which it is not possible to remove the cause. For instance, a patient may have glaucoma due to habitual tension. It is possible to relieve the patient, but permanent cure will have to depend on both the patient's emotional control, or his/her ability to relax under stressful conditions. Under such conditions, the healer may repeat the treatment at a faster interval so that the rate of healing is much faster than the rate of deterioration until the affected organ is in a very healthy state. The treatment then can be given at longer intervals to counteract deterioration due to the presence of factors causing the disease.

Before treating the patient, the healer should establish a rapport with the patient to reduce resistance. The patient should assume the receptive pose. If the patient is religious, it would be advisable to pray to make him or her more receptive. The healer should be flexible enough to adapt to different patients' needs.

Advanced Treatments

WE WILL NOW WORK with advanced techniques for treating various ailments. Some of these have already been mentioned in the intermediate section, but you will now be working with color. Please note that it is very important to wash your hands before treatment, after sweeping, after energizing, and when you are done working with each patient.

Should you encounter a situation that puzzles you and you don't know exactly what you are treating, I have provided a technique that can be effectively used in most cases.

WHAT TO DO WHEN YOU'RE NOT SURE

This information is to be used by advanced pranic healers only.

1) Apply general sweeping several times.

2) Apply localized sweeping on all vital organs.

3) Apply localized sweeping and energizing with whitish light-violet prana on all the major chakras except the spleen and meng mein chakras. Do not energize these two chakras.

4) Repeat the treatment regularly.

You can use these procedures for almost any type of ailment.

LEUKEMIA

Patients suffering from leukemia have very depleted basic and ajna chakras. The basic and meng mein chakras are overactivated but very depleted. The minor chakras in the arms and legs are also depleted. The weakening of these major and minor chakras causes the blood to become abnormal.

1) Apply general sweeping several times.

2) The meng mein chakra and basic chakra, which have been abnormally overactive for a considerable period of time, have been responsible for the abnormal increase in the production of white blood cells. Therefore, it is very important to inhibit the meng mein chakra by energizing with blue prana, and simultaneously willing these chakras to become smaller—to about three inches in diameter. Apply localized cleansing and energizing with blue prana on the meng mein chakra, and simultaneously will this overactivated chakra to become two-and-a-half inches in diameter. Rescan the meng mein chakra sideways to determine whether you have successfully inhibited this chakra.

3) Clean and energize the basic chakra with a little light whitish-green prana, then with a lot of light whitish-red prana, and with light whitish-violet prana. Cleansing and energizing this chakra would take quite some time, for it will be very depleted. This chakra controls and energizes the bones and consequently controls the production of blood.

4) Clean and energize the crown, forehead, ajna, and back head chakras with a little light whitish-green prana, then with a lot of light whitish-violet prana. Then energize the ajna chakra with light whitish-red prana.

5) Apply localized sweeping on the liver thoroughly.

6) Apply localized sweeping and energizing on the back heart, back spleen, back solar plexus, and navel chakras with a little light whitish-green prana, then with a lot of light whitish-red prana, and light whitish-violet prana.

7) Apply localized sweeping on the arms and legs. Energize the hand, elbow, armpit, as well as the sole, knee, and hip chakras with light whitish-red, and light whitish-violet prana. Visualize the pranic energy going inside the bones. The light red prana stimulates the production of red blood cells, while the light violet prana helps normalize the condition of the bones. When energizing, do not project simultaneously the light red prana and light violet prana because this is too potent and will adversely affect the condition of the patient.

Repeat the treatment three times a week for about five months or for as long as necessary. If treatment is done properly, three treatments per week is enough. Do not repeat the treatment too frequently because the patient might become overenergized and the rate of healing would be slowed down. Due to karmic factors and the debilitated condition of the patient, there is no guarantee that the patient will be completely cured. But definitely, the patient's health will be greatly improved.

Encourage the patient to become a vegetarian. Aside from the health benefits derived from a vegetarian diet, being a vegetarian is also an act of showing mercy toward the animal kingdom. Based on the law of karma, a person who shows mercy will also receive mercy. This may encourage faster healing of the patient's illness. Furthermore, instruct the patient to practice Meditation on the Twin Hearts regularly to help generate more positive karma. This meditation is described in the next chapter.

SICKLE CELL ANEMIA

1) Apply general sweeping.

2) The basic chakra is depleted, so apply localized sweeping and energizing thoroughly with light whitish-red, then with light whitish-violet prana on the basic chakra.

3) Apply localized sweeping on the legs. Then apply localized sweeping and energizing on the sole, knee and hip chakras with light whitish-red,

then with light whitish-violet prana. Visualize the pranic energy going inside the bones.

4) Apply localized sweeping on the liver.

5) Apply localized sweeping and energizing on the back heart, back spleen, back solar plexus, and navel chakras with a little light whitish-green prana, then with a lot of light whitish-red prana, and light whitish-violet prana.

6) Apply localized sweeping on the arms. Then apply localized sweeping and energizing thoroughly on the hand, elbow, and armpit chakras with light whitish-red, then with light whitish-violet prana. Visualize the pranic energy going inside the bones. Cleansing and energizing the basic chakra and the bones would gradually help normalize the condition of the blood.

7) Apply localized sweeping and energizing on the crown, forehead, ajna, and back head chakras with light whitish-violet prana.

8) Repeat the treatment three times a week for several months or for as long as necessary.

CANCER OR MALIGNANT TUMORS

A cancerous organ or part is clairvoyantly seen as dark muddy yellow and red. There is too much yellow and red prana in the affected area, resulting in the rampant growth of cancerous cells. This condition is brought about by an overactivated basic chakra, meng mein chakra, and solar plexus chakra. Although these chakras are overactivated, they are very depleted. Anger, resentment, hatred or fear activates the solar plexus chakra. The overactivated solar plexus chakra in turn activates the meng mein and basic chakras. This, in the long run, may manifest as cancer. It seems that negative emotions in the form of long-standing anger, resentment, hatred or fear is a major contributing cause of cancer.

1) Apply general sweeping several times. Many cancer patients, if not all, have blackish or darkish gray auras. The outer, health, and inner auras are all badly affected.

2) Inhibit the overactivated but depleted solar plexus, meng mein and basic chakras. This is very important in order to correct the condition causing the rapid growth of cancer cells. Apply localized sweeping and

energizing on the solar plexus chakra with green, violet and dark blue prana. Then inhibit the solar plexus chakra by willing the solar plexus chakra to become smaller (about three inches in diameter) while energizing with dark blue prana.

Apply localized sweeping and energizing thoroughly on the basic and meng mein chakras with light green prana, light whitish-violet prana, then with dark blue prana. Inhibiting the meng mein and basic chakras is done by willing these chakras to become two-and-a-half inches in diameter while energizing with dark blue prana. The solar plexus, basic and meng mein chakras usually become overactivated again after a day or two. This is why treatment has to be repeated three times a week.

3) To enhance the defense mechanism of the body, clean the bones in the arms and legs thoroughly by applying localized sweeping. Energize the sole, knee, and hip chakras with light whitish-violet prana, and visualize pranic energy going inside the bones. Energize the hand, elbow, and armpit chakras with light violet and visualize the pranic energy going inside the bones.

4) Clean, energize and activate the crown, forehead, ajna, back head, and throat chakras with light green, light blue and light violet prana. When energizing with light violet prana, will the crown, forehead, ajna, and throat chakras to become bigger (about five or six inches in diameter) and the back head chakra to about two inches in diameter. This is to activate the upper chakras in order to produce more green, blue, and violet prana, which have neutralizing effects on cancer cells.

5) Clean the front and back heart chakras thoroughly. Energize the back heart chakra with light whitish-violet prana and simultaneously will the heart chakra to become five or six inches in diameter; this will help the patient experience a sense of inner peace.

6) Apply cleansing on the affected parts. This is done by applying localized sweeping on the affected part about one to two hundred times. This will partially or completely relieve the patient of pain. Be sure to wash your hands regularly while cleansing. You must remember that the affected part is very dirty, congested, and filled with dark muddy red and yellow pranas. Energize the affected part with dark blue prana for about fifteen minutes in order to inhibit the growth of cancer cells and to localize them. Also inhibit the affected chakra which is overactivated. Energize the affected part with your finger with dark green prana, then with dark orange prana about five minutes each. Visualize the pranic energy coming out as laser-

like and as thin as the tip of a ball point. The dark green prana, and dark orange prana have to be projected in a very concentrated form to give it sufficient potency to partially disintegrate the cancer cells. Do not use orange prana on delicate organs.

7) Repeat the treatment three times a week for five months, or for as long as necessary. The treatment should not be done too frequently because the patient might be overenergized and the healing process might be slowed down.

Encourage the patient to become a vegetarian. Aside from the benefits derived from a vegetarian diet, being a vegetarian is an act of showing mercy toward the animal kingdom. Based on the law of karma, a person who shows mercy will also in turn receive mercy. This encourages faster healing of the illness. Furthermore, instruct the patient to practice Meditation on Twin Hearts regularly to help generate more positive karma.

The following are the benefits derived by cancer patients from this form of healing: the intense pain will be gradually reduced after several treatments; the energy level of the patient will be increased and the patient will feel much stronger after several treatments. The appetite will improve; the growth of the cancer cells will be reduced if not stopped; and the cancer cells will be gradually and partially destroyed. For terminal cancer patients, pranic healing will enable them to die in peace and with dignity.

Some cancer patients cannot be healed for a number of reasons. The patient's body may have already been badly damaged by potent drugs. The cancer cells may have already spread; or the body is extremely weak and its capacity to absorb and retain pranic energy has greatly diminished. Sometimes organ(s) have been so badly damaged that they are beyond repair. And last, the ailment could be of karmic origin. Because of these factors, some cancer patients will be partially or completely relieved, their health improved, and their life prolonged, but only a few will be completely cured.

VENEREAL DISEASES

1) Apply general sweeping with light whitish-green prana several times.

2) Apply localized sweeping on the sex chakra and the sex organs. Energize them thoroughly with greenish-blue prana, then violet prana. Green, blue and violet prana have strong disinfecting properties. Do not use red prana for it activates the germs, causing the disease to become worse. It

is also not advisable to use yellow and orange prana, for the former may stimulate the growth of the germs, while the latter would cause the germs to spread.

3) Clean and energize all the other affected parts thoroughly with green, blue, and violet prana.

4) Clean and energize the navel, solar plexus, throat, ajna, forehead, and crown chakras with light green, light blue and light violet prana.

5) To stimulate the defense mechanism of the body, apply localized sweeping and energizing thoroughly on the sole, knee, hip, armpit, elbow, and hand chakras with light whitish-violet prana, and visualize the pranic energy penetrating the bones.

6) Apply localized sweeping on the depleted basic chakra. Do not energize it because if it is overenergized, it may tend to activate the venereal germs and would make the condition worse. Also do not use the master healing technique for the same reason.

CYSTS

1) Apply localized sweeping on the affected part.

2) Energize the affected part with light blue prana for about five breathing cycles, whitish-green prana for ten breathing cycles and with whitish-orange prana for ten breathing cycles. This is to disintegrate the cyst. Repeat the treatment three times a week.

3) After one or two weeks, energize the affected part with green prana and orange prana, then with light whitish-yellow prana for one breathing cycle. This is to facilitate the removal of the disintegrated matter.

SEXUAL IMPOTENCE

1) Clean and energize the basic, sex and navel chakras with light whitish-red prana. The navel chakra, to a certain extent, energizes the sexual organs. Energizing the navel chakra also increases the general energy level of the body.

2) Apply localized sweeping thoroughly on the front and back solar plexus chakras. Energize them with light whitish-blue prana.

Do not use this technique if the patient is suffering from, or has a history of, sexually transmitted diseases.

IRREGULAR MENSTRUATION AND DYSMENORRHEA

1) Scan the affected area and apply localized sweeping on the sex chakra, navel chakra, basic chakra, and the lower portion of the spine.

2) Energize the sex and navel chakras with light whitish-orange prana for five breathing cycles for each chakra.

3) Energize the basic chakra with light red prana for four breathing cycles.

BACKACHE OR INJURED BACK

1) Apply localized sweeping on the spine and on the affected part.

2) Energize the affected part with light whitish-green prana for four breathing cycles, next with light whitish-blue prana for four breathing cycles, and then with light whitish-red prana for four breathing cycles. The master healing technique may be applied to accelerate the healing process.

DIABETES

1) Apply general sweeping.

2) Clean the front and back solar plexus chakras. Energize the pancreas through the back solar plexus chakra; first, with light whitish-green prana, second, with light whitish-blue prana, and third, with light violet prana.

This is to heal the pancreas so that it will normalize its production of insulin.

3) Scan the ajna chakra. If there is pranic congestion, apply localized sweeping and energize with light violet prana. Instruct mentally or verbally the patient's ajna chakra to normalize the production of insulin. Repeat the treatment two times a week.

ASTHMA

1) Apply general sweeping several times.

2) Apply localized sweeping on the throat chakra and on the secondary throat minor chakra. The secondary throat minor chakra is located on the lower soft portion of the throat. Energize them with light green prana for one breathing cycle, then with light whitish-red prana for four or more breathing cycles for each chakra.

3) Apply localized sweeping on the lungs and on the back heart chakra. Energize the lungs through the back heart chakra with light green prana for one breathing cycle, then with light whitish-red prana for ten breathing cycles. Clean and energize the solar plexus chakra with light whitish-red prana for five breathing cycles. This will give the patient immediate relief.

4) To gradually and completely heal the patient, energize the ajna chaka with light violet prana and basic chakras with light whitish-red prana.

5) To improve the quality of the blood produced, the bones in the body have to be cleansed and energized. Apply localized sweeping and simultaneously energize the spinal column with light whitish-red prana several times.

6) Apply localized sweeping and simultaneously visualize your hand going into the bones of the arms and legs. Energize the bones in the arms through the hand and armpit chakras with light whitish-red prana for five breathing cycles for each chakra. Visualize the light red pranic energy going into the bones in the arms, the shoulder blades and the chest bones. Energize the bones in the legs through the sole chakras and the hip chakras with light red prana for five breathing cycles for each chakra. Visualize the light red pranic energy going into the hip bones and the bones in the legs. This

technique is very effective in treating asthmatic cases. The purpose of this pranic treatment is to improve the quality of the blood produced, thereby gradually making the patient immune to irritants.

7) Repeat the treatment two or three times a week.

LUNG INFECTION/TUBERCULOSIS

1) Apply general sweeping.

2) Apply localized sweeping on the lungs and on the back heart chakra.

3) First, energize the back heart chakra and the lungs with light whitish-green prana for five breathing cycles, then with light whitish-blue prana for five breathing cycles. This is to cleanse and disinfect the lungs. If the infection is severe, energize with light violet prana for ten breathing cycles.

4) For strengthening and eliminating effects, energize the lungs with light whitish-orange prana for four breathing cycles, then with light whitish-red prana for three breathing cycles.

5) Energize the solar plexus chakra with light whitish-red prana for seven breathing cycles to energize the lower lungs and the entire physical body.

6) If the nose and throat are affected then they should be treated also.

7) For patients suffering from a severe lung infection or tuberculosis, apply the master healing technique. This will greatly accelerate the healing process. With the use of the master healing technique, it is possible to completely heal a patient with tuberculosis within a month or two. Repeat the entire treatment twice a week. If the patient is very weak and in critical condition, treatments should be given at faster intervals.

Since the back heart chakra is so closely related to the front heart chakra, malfunctioning of the lungs may severely affect the heart and vice versa. In healing patients with lung problems, it is important to also scan the front heart chakra.

SINUSITIS AND STUFFY NOSE

1) Apply general sweeping several times.

2) Apply localized sweeping and energizing on the forehead chakra, the ajna chakra and on the root of the nose with light green prana for five breathing cycles, and with light whitish-blue prana for seven breathing cycles for each chakra.

3) Cleanse and energize the right and left nostril minor chakras with light green prana for two breathing cycles and with light blue prana for two breathing cycles for each minor chakra.

4) Energize the back head chakra with white prana for three breathing cycles. Usually the relief is very fast. Check the temples, the throat and the lungs. Repeat the treatment twice a week.

COUGH

1) Apply general sweeping several times.

2) Clean and energize the throat chakra and the secondary throat chakra with light green prana for three breathing cycles, with light whitish-orange prana for two breathing cycles and with light whitish-blue prana for four breathing cycles.

3) Energize the solar plexus chakra with white prana for seven breathing cycles. If the nose and lungs are affected, then they should be treated also.

NEARSIGHTEDNESS, FARSIGHTEDNESS, ASTIGMATISM, CROSS-EYES, WALLEYES, CATARACT

1) Apply localized sweeping on the brain, the ajna chakra, the eyes and the temple chakras.

2) Energize the eyes through the ajna chakra with light whitish-green prana for five breathing cycles. This is to clean and loosen the used-up prana in the minute nadis of the eyes. Energize the eyes with light whitish-

yellow prana for one breathing cycle. Apply localized sweeping on the eyes.

3) Energize the eyes with light whitish-violet prana for five breathing cycles. This is to strengthen the eyes. Energize the eyes with light blue prana for two breathing cycles. This is to stabilize the projected prana and to give pliability or flexibility to the parts of the eyes.

4) Energize the back head chakra with white prana for four breathing cycles and visualize the pranic energy going into the eyes.

Repeat the treatment two to three times a week. The patient should avoid wearing eyeglasses for the duration of the treatment as this tends to neutralize the effects of the treatments. If the preceding conditions can be followed, it is quite likely that the patient may be completely healed within three months. The rate of healing will depend on the patient's age, the condition of the patient's eyes, and the proficiency of the healer.

Once the patient has been healed, he or she should not overuse the eyes and should go back for periodic treatments, especially if he or she feels the eyes weakening. This is just like visiting your dentist once or twice a year.

GLAUCOMA

1) Clean the eyes, the temples and the ajna chakra. Energize the eyes through the ajna chakra with whitish-green prana, then with light whitish-blue prana. Apply localized sweeping and energizing alternately until there is substantial relief.

2) Energize the eyes through the ajna chakra with light violet prana for seven breathing cycles to regenerate the eyes.

3) Energize the back head chakra with white prana for four breathing cycles and visualize the pranic energy going into the eyes.

4) The treatment should be done three times a week for a month or two even if the patient does not feel any pain or discomfort.

Do not use orange prana in treating eye problems. This may result in irreversible eye damage!

FLOATER

Clean the ajna chakra, the eyes and the temple minor chakras. Energize the eyes through the ajna chakra with white prana or with light whitish-green prana for ten breathing cycles. Repeat the treatment three times a week.

EYE INFECTIONS

1) Since it is clairvoyantly observed that some patients suffering from eye infections have holes in their outer auras, apply general sweeping. A portion of the health aura droops and the health rays are entangled. Very often the application of general sweeping makes the difference between a rapid rate of healing and a much slower rate of healing.

2) Apply localized sweeping and energize with light whitish-green prana for four breathing cycles, then with light whitish-blue prana for seven breathing cycles. Use light violet prana if the infection is severe.

3) Cleanse and energize the back head chakra with white prana. Visualize the eyes being energized and becoming brighter.

4) If there is ulceration, energize with light violet prana for five breathing cycles and then with light whitish-greenish yellow prana for five breathing cycles in order to accelerate the healing of the wound.

5) Energize the navel chakra, the solar plexus chakra, the hand chakras, and the sole chakras to strengthen the body's defense system.

CHRONIC RED EYES

Clean and energize the eyes through the ajna chakra with light whitish-blue prana for ten breathing cycles. Apply treatments three times a week.

ACUTE APPENDICITIS

1) Apply general sweeping several times.

2) Apply localized sweeping on the solar plexus chakra, the navel chakra, the appendix and the entire abdominal area.

3) Apply localized sweeping on the entire spine.

4) Energize the front solar plexus chakra and the navel chakra with light green prana for ten breathing cycles for each chakra, and with light blue prana for ten breathing cycles for each chakra. Visualize the prana going to the appendix. This is very important since the solar plexus and the navel chakras control and energize the large intestines, including the appendix. That is why a person suffering from acute appendicitis initially feels pain in the solar plexus area.

5) Energize the hand and the sole chakras with light violet prana to strengthen the body's defense system.

Repeat the treatment once every one-and-a-half hours for the next six hours or until the condition has stabilized. When the condition has stabilized, you may repeat the entire treatment twice a day for the next few days. Do not energize with orange prana because it may accelerate the rupturing of the inflamed appendix. The patient should be hospitalized during the treatments so that his condition can be closely monitored by medical doctors, and emergency surgery can be performed if the situation requires it.

This treatment is used for healing acute appendicitis that is about one day old. If the patient has already been in pain for several days before approaching a pranic healer, it is better if he will be operated on since the risk of rupture of the inflamed appendix is greater. If you are not experienced at diagnosis, don't work on the patient until he or she is in the hospital. However, you can certainly assist the patient on the way to the doctor.

Patients who have been recently healed should avoid heavy or strenuous exercises for the next few months. Heavy meals should also be avoided. They should have daily bowel movements and should go back for further treatment if they experience slight pain in the appendix area.

For treating chronic appendicitis, just energize the solar plexus and navel chakras with light whitish-green prana, and light whitish-blue prana.

HEART AILMENTS

There are many types of heart ailments. Heart ailments may manifest as the heart's muscle failure due to clotting or obstruction in the heart arteries, as heart infection, as malfunctioning of the heart valves, as heart congestion either of the left or right heart, as holes in the dividing wall between the left and the right heart, as an irregular beating of the heart, or as a heart enlargement.

In pranic healing, these problems manifest as either pranic heart congestion or depletion or both simultaneously. With pranic heart congestion, the emphasis should be on localized sweeping. With pranic heart depletion, the emphasis should be on energizing. Apply localized sweeping on the front and back heart chakras, and on the solar plexus chakra. In treating heart ailments, white prana or light green prana and light red prana are usually used in energizing. Orange prana is not used here because of its possible damaging effect on the heart.

1) Scan the heart thoroughly. The heart must be scanned with one or two fingers to locate the small trouble spots. To help you locate these, ask the patient what specific spots hurt.

2) Apply general sweeping. Clean the front heart chakra thoroughly. The small spots with pranic depletion must be cleansed thoroughly with the use of your fingers. Visualize white light or prana coming out of your fingers and removing the diseased bioplasmic matter.

3) Clean the front and back heart chakras and the front and back solar plexus chakras.

4) Energize the heart through the back heart chakra with white prana for ten breathing cycles. Visualize the heart and the front heart chakra as very bright and healthy.

5) Or energize the heart with light whitish-green prana for seven breathing cycles and then with light whitish-red prana for five breathing cycles. Light green prana breaks down diseased bioplasmic matter and also directly and indirectly causes the physical obstruction to dissolve. Light red prana has a dilating and strengthening effect on the heart.

6) Energize the solar plexus chakra with white prana for five breathing cycles. Rescan the heart to determine whether it has been properly and thoroughly treated. Get feedback from the patient.

7) For an inflamed heart, clean and energize the heart with light whitish-green prana for five breathing cycles, and with light whitish-blue prana for seven breathing cycles.

8) For a heart with a defective valve, or with physical wounds or holes, energize with light whitish-green-violet prana for nine breathing cycles, with light green-yellow prana for three breathing cycles, and with light whitish-red prana for three breathing cycles.

9) Clean and energize the basic and navel chakras with white prana. This will strengthen the body and further accelerate the rate of healing.

The treatment should be given at least three times a week. If the patient cannot be disturbed, energize the heart by visualizing the back of the patient in front of your palm. Pranic healing is very effective for heart ailments. Usually the patient fully recovers in a short time.

HIGH BLOOD PRESSURE

Although dietary habits and tension are major factors contributing to high blood pressure, this ailment manifests as pranic congestion and overactivation of the meng mein chakra. Sometimes the meng mein chakra is overactivated and depleted. I experienced high blood pressure when I was experimenting on activating and energizing the basic, meng mein, and spleen chakras. The etheric body (or bioplasmic body), when seen clairvoyantly, was very bright and glaring. Because of the extremely high pranic energy level, the body felt quite weak and concentration was difficult.

If the basic chakra is depleted, then there is general pranic depletion of the body. If the basic chakra is quite active, then there is general pranic congestion of the body.

1) Scan the whole body. Scan the meng mein chakra frontally to determine the degree of pranic congestion and then scan it sideways to determine the size or degree of overactivation. An overactivated meng mein chakra sometimes has a diameter of five inches or more while the other chakras are only about three to four inches in diameter.

2) Apply general sweeping several times.

3) Apply localized sweeping thoroughly on the back head area, spine, and the front and back solar plexus, meng mein, and basic chakras. In most cases, cleansing alone will greatly relieve the patient.

4) Clean the meng mein chakra thoroughly. Inhibit the meng mein chakra by energizing with blue prana, coupled with a strong intention of inhibiting the degree of activity of the meng mein chakra and visualizing it getting smaller. Visualize the meng mein chakra as becoming smaller to about three inches in diameter and also dimmer or not too bright. Rescan the meng mein chakra. Once the meng mein chakra is successfully inhibited, the blood pressure will gradually drop. Repeat this procedure after one or two hours since there is a big possibility that the meng mein chakra will become overactivated again.

5) The solar plexus chakra is usually congested and over-activated. Energize the front and back solar plexus chakras with light whitish-blue prana and apply more localized sweeping.

6) Some of the major head chakras are congested while some are depleted. Clean and energize the crown, forehead, ajna and back head chakras with white prana.

7) The heart is usually affected. It may be congested or depleted, or both. Apply pranic treatment on the heart.

Repeat the treatment three times a week. Send the patient to a doctor for complementary treatment.

ARTERIOSCLEROSIS (HARDENING OF THE ARTERIES)

1) Apply general sweeping.

2) Energize the ajna chakra with light whitish-green prana for three breathing cycles, with light whitish-red prana for three breathing cycles, and with light whitish-blue prana for three breathing cycles.

3) Do the same with the back heart chakra, the solar plexus chakra and the basic chakra. Repeat the treatment twice a week.

ARTHRITIS OR RHEUMATISM

Arthritis and rheumatism are very broad terms used in relation to muscle pain and disorder of the joints. Disorder of the joints may be caused by solidification of liquid calcium, accumulation of urates, chalky salts of uric acid, or the degeneration of the protective shock-absorbing cartilage in the joints.

Arthritis or rheumatism manifests as pranic depletion of the minor chakras on the arms and legs and partial pranic depletion in some major chakras.

Minor chakras related to the arms are the finger chakras, hand chakras, elbow chakras, armpit chakras, back neck chakra, secondary throat chakra, and nipple chakras. Patients with joint ailments in the arms may have depleted nipple chakras, or back neck chakra and secondary throat chakra. Sometimes, it is necessary to energize the tip of the affected finger.

Minor chakras related to the legs are the toe chakras, sole .chakras, knee chakras, hip chakras, and perineum chakra. Sometimes it is necessary to energize the tip of the affected toe.

Major chakras related to joint ailments are the basic chakra, meng mein chakra, kidneys, sex chakra, navel chakra, solar plexus chakra, spleen chakra, and ajna chakra.

Sometimes patients with heart ailments or with high blood pressure may have difficulty moving or raising the left or right arms. So please take note, some patients with this ailment may be susceptible to stroke.

Orange and red pranas are used in treating mild arthritis or rheumatism. For simple muscle pain or mild. arthritis in the joints, apply localized sweeping and energize with light whitish-orange prana for five breathing cycles and then with light whitish-red prana for five breathing cycles. It most cases, the relief is immediate. The patient may feel a cold energy or current being expelled from the affected part.

1) Apply general sweeping thoroughly.

2) The affected parts in severe arthritis or rheumatism are very inflamed and depleted. Apply localized sweeping on the entire affected arm or leg. Clean and energize the painful joints with greenish-blue prana for ten breathing cycles. Then with light violet prana also for ten breathing cycles. The use of too much orange and red prana is not advisable for it may aggravate the condition. Thorough cleansing or sweeping is very important.

3) To strengthen and improve circulation, energize the affected part with light whitish-red prana for two breathing cycles.

4) If the arms or fingers are affected, apply localized sweeping and energizing with light green prana, then with a lot of light violet prana on

the armpit, elbow, and hand chakras. If the fingers are affected, apply localized sweeping and energizing on fingers, joints, and tips of the fingers with light green prana, then with a lot of light violet prana. With patients suffering from arthritis of the fingers, the armpit, elbow, and hand chakras have to be treated because they are filled with diseased energy.

5) If the leg(s) or toes are affected, apply localized sweeping and energizing on the hip, knee, and sole chakras with light green prana, then with a lot of light violet prana. If the toes are affected, the hip, knee and sole chakras have to be treated because they are filled with diseased energy.

6) The basic chakra controls and energizes the skeletal and muscular systems of the body. In cases of severe arthritis and rheumatism, the basic chakra is very depleted. Therefore it is very important to highly energize this chakra. To effect a more lasting cure, apply localized sweeping on the liver; then clean and energize the basic chakra, sex, solar plexus, navel, and spleen chakra with a little whitish-green prana, and then with a lot of whitish-red prana, and light whitish-violet prana. You may also use the master healing technique. This will produce rapid relief when done properly. With patients suffering from hypertension, do not energize the spleen chakra, and do not use the master healing technique.

7) For milder rheumatoid arthritis, apply treatments twice a week for one month. The patient will experience substantial relief and improvement after two or three sessions. For more serious rheumatoid arthritis, apply treatment three times a week for two months or as long as necessary. Most patients will experience substantial relief and improvement in a week or two.

8) In cases of severe gout, the affected part should be treated three to five times a day for three days or more. The basic chakra, sex, solar plexus, and navel chakras should be treated twice a day for three days or more. Apply localized sweeping thoroughly on the meng mein chakra and the kidneys. Then energize the kidneys directly (without energizing the meng mein chakra) with light whitish-green prana, then with light whitish-red, and with light whitish-violet prana. This is to strengthen the kidneys and improve its eliminative function. It would be helpful if the patient could do something to clean the large intestines. This will greatly accelerate the rate of healing. Also the patient is expected to watch his or her diet.

NEW AND OLD SPRAINS

1) Apply localized sweeping to the affected part and on the affected minor chakras.

2) Energize with light orange-red prana for seven breathing cycles or until the pain completely disappears. Energizing the affected part directly is quite effective in producing instant relief. Very often, the relief for a new sprain is instantaneous and permanent as long as the patient does not immediately overexert the treated part.

3) For an old sprain, use light greenish-red prana. It may require several treatments to produce permanent relief.

HOW TO STRENGTHEN THE LEGS

1) Activate and energize the basic and perineum minor chakras with light red prana for seven breathing cycles for each chakra. This will cause an increase in the flow of pranic energy from the basic chakra to the legs.

2) Energize the sex chakra with white prana for seven breathing cycles. A substantial portion of prana from the sex chakra automatically goes down to the legs.

3) Apply localized sweeping to the legs with whitish-orange prana.

4) Energize the sole, knee and hip minor chakras on the leg or legs with light red prana for five breathing cycles for each chakra. This entire pranic treatment can be used to heal weak legs and paralysis of the legs. If the paralysis is localized or does not involve the brain or the spine, then the recovery will be fast.

HOW TO STRENGTHEN THE ARMS

1) Apply localized sweeping on the arms.

2) Clean the armpit minor chakra by raising the arm of the patient and by applying localized sweeping on the armpit. This is very important.

Difficulty in raising the arm could be caused by pranic congestion or depletion of the armpit minor chakra. Cleansing and energizing this minor chakra usually brings instant relief.

3) Energize the hand chakras, the elbow chakras and the nipple chakras with light red prana for five breathing cycles per chakra. This pranic treatment can be used to treat arm paralysis if the cause is of local origin. A person with arm ailments, like old sprains, usually has depleted nipple chakras. You may energize and strengthen the entire arm through the nipple minor chakras. Visualize light red prana going into the nipple minor chakra and to the entire arm.

FEVER

1) Apply general sweeping several times with whitish-green prana.

2) To clean, soothe, cool and disinfect the entire body, clean and energize the front solar plexus chakra with light whitish-green prana for four breathing cycles and then with light whitish-blue prana for four breathing cycles.

3) To eliminate and expel diseased bioplasmic matter, toxins, and germs from the body, energize the front solar plexus chakra with light whitish-orange prana for three breathing cycles.

4) Energize the navel chakra, the hand chakras and the sole chakras with white prana for five breathing cycles for each chakra.

5) If the throat and/or the lungs are affected, then they should also be treated. The entire treatment may be repeated after one or two hours.

6) With infants or children just use white prana for the entire treatment. General sweeping should be emphasized and energizing should be done gently and gradually.

ACUTE PANCREATITIS

Acute pancreatitis is a severe inflammation of the pancreas. The patient feels intense pain in the solar plexus area and the back of it. Fever, chills, cold sweats, vomiting and headaches are experienced. The patient is in a state of severe shock.

This manifests as a serious imbalance of the solar plexus chakra and the entire etheric body (or bioplasmic body) is affected.

1) Apply general sweeping several times. There will be noticeable relief after applying general sweeping.

2) Apply localized sweeping on the solar plexus chakra and energize it with whitish-blue prana for twelve breathing cycles. Blue prana soothes the pain and inhibits the pancreas from excreting more digestive juice. Avoid using yellow prana or orange prana or both. This may stimulate or trigger the pancreas to produce more juice, thereby making the patient worse.

Apply the treatment three times once every three hours on the first few days. The patient may be greatly or fully relieved on the first day. The rate of healing is usually very fast.

HEPATITIS

Inflammation of the liver, or hepatitis, could be caused by a virus, toxins, or a prolonged period of excessive alcohol intake. Inflammation manifests as malfunctioning of the solar plexus chakra and pranic congestion or depletion of the liver.

1) Apply general sweeping several times.

2) Clean and energize the solar plexus chakra and the liver. The liver is divided into left and right parts. Sometimes, a portion of the liver may be pranically congested while the other part may be pranically depleted. To soothe, disinfect, and clean the liver, energize the front solar plexus chakra and the liver with light green prana for ten breathing cycles, with light blue prana for ten breathing cycles and with light violet prana for ten breathing cycles. If the inflammation is caused by toxins, more green prana should be used to facilitate the breaking down of the toxins.

3) In acute hepatitis, or if the inflammation is severe, the rate of pranic consumption is very fast. To produce rapid healing, the liver and the solar plexus chakra should be treated once every two hours for the next eight hours. Repeat the treatment twice a day for the next few days.

4) To strengthen the body and to further increase the rate of healing, clean and energize the navel chakra, the spleen chakra, the hand chakras and the sole chakras. This master healing technique should not be used on patients with cirrhosis of the liver. If the kidneys are also affected, visualize the prana going to the kidneys when energizing the meng mein chakra. The kidneys should be cleansed before energizing.

5) If the patient has a bloated abdomen and legs, clean and energize the navel chakra, and the abdomen. Clean and energize the sole chakras.

Liver ailments should be treated as early as possible. If the patient is young and the liver ailment is treated at its early stage, then the rate of healing would be very fast; but if the patient is old and has had the liver ailment for quite a time already, then the rate of healing would likely be slow and difficult. The patient may feel a certain degree of improvement but full recovery takes a lot of time. In some cases, it may not be possible to cure the patient at all.

GALLSTONES

1) Apply localized sweeping on the front solar plexus chakra and the gallbladder.

2) To soothe, energize the gallbladder through the front solar plexus chakra with light blue prana for four breathing cycles.

3) Energize with light green prana for seven breathing cycles, and with light orange prana for seven breathing cycles to facilitate the dissolving of the deposits. To facilitate the gradual removal of the disintegrated stones, energize with whitish-yellow prana for one breathing cycle.

4) Apply the treatment once a day. The patient may be relieved completely on the first or second treatment but it should be continued until the stones are completely dissolved. Western medicine or Chinese herbal medicine should preferably be taken to supplement the treatment.

PEPTIC ULCERS

Peptic ulcers are an ulceration of the stomach or of the duodenum lining. Ulceration of the stomach lining is called gastric ulcers, while ulceration of the duodenum lining is called duodenal ulcers. Peptic ulcers manifest as malfunctioning of the solar plexus chakra and the stomach minor chakra. You would treat a mild gastric or duodenal ulcer as follows:

1) Scan the front solar plexus chakra and the abdominal area.

2) Apply localized sweeping on the front and back solar plexus chakras, on the affected area, and energize with white prana or with light blue prana. The relief is usually instantaneous for mild cases. Apply treatment twice a week.

For severe cases, you would do the following:

1) Apply localized sweeping.

2) Energize the solar plexus chakra and the affected area with light blue prana for seven breathing cycles, with light whitish-violet prana for ten breathing cycles. Visualizing the wound as healing would also be helpful. Apply treatment three times a week.

3) To accelerate the healing process, use the master healing technique.

HERNIAS

A hernia is a bulging out or a protrusion of the lower abdomen due to the weakened or ruptured abdominal wall. There are many types of hernias. In umbilical hernia, which is common in babies, the protrusion occurs in the navel area; in incisional hernia, the bulge occurs in the abdominal scar area; in inguinal hernia, the protrusion occurs in the area where the thigh joins the abdomen and may tend to go into the scrotum.

1) Scan the affected area, the navel chakra, the sex chakra, and the basic chakra.

2) Energize the basic chakra with light red prana.

3) Apply localized sweeping on the affected part, on the navel chakra, and on the sex chakra. These two chakras are partially depleted. Energize the navel chakra and the sex chakra with white prana and visualize the pranic energy going to the affected part. Energize the affected part directly with light greenish-yellow prana, then with light whitish-blue prana.

4) If the perineum is affected, clean and energize it with greenish-red prana.

5) Repeat the treatment three times a week. It may take several months for the patient to be completely healed.

A hernia should be treated as early as possible. It may develop into a strangulated hernia if the hole is quite small, thereby blocking the flow of blood, and gangrene may occur.

STONES IN THE URINARY SYSTEM

Stones may occur in the kidneys, ureter and bladder. They may cause cuts, inflammation and may block the flow of urine.

1) Scan the meng mein chakra, the kidneys, the sex chakra, the bladder, the ureter, and the lower abdominal area.

2) Apply localized sweeping on the meng mein chakra, kidneys and the sex chakra. To soothe and disinfect the affected kidney or kidneys, energize with light blue prana for seven breathing cycles.

3) To gradually disintegrate the obstruction, energize the kidneys directly with light green prana, then with light orange prana. With infants, children, and older people, energizing has to be shortened. Use only light whitish-green prana. Do not use orange prana because it may cause the meng mein chakra to become overactivated which would result in high blood pressure. Should this happen, inhibit the meng mein chakra with the use of blue prana. (See instructions for treatment of hypertension.)

4) If the obstruction is in the ureter, energize the kidneys and the sex chakra. Also energize the affected part directly.

5) Apply the same treatment for stones in the bladder. You may also use the "double energizing" technique on the affected parts directly. Repeat the treatment once or twice a day for the next one or two weeks. Although the patient may be relieved after the first treatment, several treatments still have to be given until the obstruction has been completely removed. Chinese herbal medicine or Western medicine may be taken to supplement pranic treatment.

For infants, children, and older people, just energize the kidneys directly without passing through the meng mein chakra. Overenergizing the meng mein chakra or energizing the basic and meng mein chakras may cause severe high blood pressure.

Modern medical treatment and equipment that can quickly and safely disintegrate the stones in the kidneys are available but pranic healing is still required to prevent or reduce the possibility of stone formation in the urinary system in the future.

INFLAMMATION OF THE URINARY SYSTEM

Inflammation of the bladder or kidney could be caused by infections, toxins, and stones.

1) Apply general sweeping on the entire body.

2) Apply localized sweeping on the meng mein chakra and on the kidneys.

3) To soothe and disinfect the kidneys, energize the kidneys directly with light whitish-green prana for five breathing cycles, then with light whitish-blue prana for ten breathing cycles. Apply pranic treatment three times a week.

4) To soothe, disinfect, and strengthen the bladder, apply the same pranic treatment on the bladder through the sex chakra.

5) To facilitate the elimination of fluids in the body, energize the kidneys directly with light yellow-orange prana.

As mentioned earlier, infants, children, and older people should be energized through the kidneys directly without passing through the meng mein chakra. Overenergizing the meng mein chakra or energizing the basic and meng mein chakras of infants, children, and older people may cause severe high blood pressure.

DEAFNESS

There are several causes for deafness, and pranic treatment for each type of deafness is more or less the same. Deafness manifests as malfunctioning of the ear minor chakra and there is usually slight pranic depletion on the back head minor chakra. This is seen as muddy orange on the ear minor chakra. It may manifest as pranic depletion or congestion or both simultaneously. A normal ear chakra appears as light red. In acupuncture, the ear is used as a source chakra for red prana to treat ailments in the other parts of the body.

I have encountered a strange case in which a woman patient suffered a bad fall on her basic chakra area when she was still a young child. When seen clairvoyantly, one half of the basic chakra was relatively all right while the other half was quite depleted. This occurs very rarely. The root of the basic chakra was slightly off-center. She was partially deaf in the right ear, the right eye was worse than the left eye, the right breast was smaller than the left one, and the right leg was shorter than the left. The sex chakra was also malfunctioning. Obviously, if her ailments were to be gradually cured, the basic chakra had to be normalized. The basic chakra was cleansed and energized. By the use of the will, the root of the basic chakra was gradually centered. Spinal adjustment was also applied.

1) For slight deafness, apply localized sweeping on the ear minor chakra and on the back head chakra. Very light orange prana is used in treating mild deafness due to fluid in the middle ear cavity.

2) Energize the affected ear with light whitish-green prana for three breathing cycles, and with very light whitish-orange prana for two breathing cycles. This should be done only by experienced pranic healers.

3) Apply localized sweeping on the back head chakra and energize with white prana for five breathing cycles. Visualize the prana going to the affected ear. The back head chakra plays an important role in energizing the entire head area including the eyes and ears. Do not overenergize the back head chakra since the projected prana is localized in the head area.

4) For severe deafness, apply the same treatment as the preceding case. Use light violet or greenish-violet and greenish-yellow pranas. Energize the affected ear with light greenish-violet prana for twelve breathing cycles, with light greenish-yellow prana for three breathing cycles. This treatment can be used for a ruptured eardrum or nerve deafness.

Most patients may experience immediate and substantial improvement with their hearing. Sometimes, the treated ear hears better than the other normal ear but this improvement is usually temporary in most cases. Treatments have to be repeated once every two or three days until the healing is complete.

HEADACHES, TOOTHACHES, STOMACHACHES, CONSTIPATION AND DIARRHEA

For headaches and toothaches, apply localized sweeping and energizing on the affected area and affected chakras with light green prana, then light blue prana. Many patients can be instantly relieved just by sweeping only. For abdominal problems, the solar plexus and navel chakras should be treated. For gas pains, use white prana. For diarrhea, use whitish-green prana, and whitish-blue prana or greenish-blue prana. Do not use orange prana on diarrhea patients. Cleansing or localized sweeping should be emphasized. For constipation, energize the front solar plexus chakra and the navel chakra with light orange prana or yellow prana. If the large intestine has been weakened, energize it with light red prana.

INSOMNIA

1) Apply general sweeping with whitish-blue prana. Blue prana is soothing and sleep inducing. Do not apply general sweeping with greenish-blue prana because with some patients it may have disruptive effects.

2) If the patient is depleted, energize the solar plexus chakra, the navel chakra, the sole chakras and the hand chakras with white prana.

3) If the crown chakra or the other head chakras are affected, clean and energize them with whitish-blue prana.

CONCUSSION

For fresh concussion, cleanse and energize the affected part with light blue, light green, and light orange pranas. Repeat the treatment several times for the next few hours. For an old or blackened concussion, energize the affected part with green, orange and red pranas. Do not use orange prana on the head area.

FAINTING

Energize the navel chakra with white prana to revive the person. A portion of the prana will go to the solar plexus then to the head area. Simultaneously the spleen chakra is automatically energized, which in turn energizes the other chakras. This is one of the safest techniques.

You may also energize the back head chakra which will energize the entire head area. This method is faster but there is the possibility of overenergizing the entire head area. This technique should be used with caution.

DROWNING

First aid measures should be simultaneously applied with the pranic treatment. Energize intensely the back solar plexus chakra and the back heart chakra with light red prana. If the subject is still not revived, then use the master healing technique.

FOOD POISONING

Clean the abdomen and energize the solar plexus chakra and the navel chakra with greenish-blue prana. Do not use orange prana if the treated area is near a delicate organ. The relief is usually fast. If the condition worsens, bring the patient to the hospital immediately.

SKIN BLEMISHES

Clean and energize the affected skin with light green prana, with light orange prana, then with light red prana. Do not use orange prana if the treated area is near a delicate organ. The surrounding skin area should also be cleansed and energized to facilitate the healing process.

EPILEPSY

1) To alleviate an epileptic condition or to substantially reduce the frequency of epileptic attacks, apply general sweeping.

2) Clean the entire head area.

3) Energize the ajna, the forehead, crown, and the back head chakra (which is located at the center of the back of the head) with whitish-green prana for two breathing cycles and with whitish-violet prana for five breathing cycles for each chakra. You should visualize the right brain and the left brain being equalized. With an epileptic patient, one side of the brain is partially depleted while the other side is partially congested.

4) Clean and energize the solar plexus chakra and the heart chakra with whitish-pink prana for five breathing cycles for each chakra. The front heart chakra should be energized through the back heart chakra.

5) Check the entire spine. Apply pranic treatment twice a week for the next several months.

SUMMARY

Cleansing and energizing are the basic principles in pranic healing. Diseased bioplasmic matter or diseased etheric matter are removed from the affected chakras and parts. The affected chakras and parts are energized with prana. By healing or by repeated treatments on the bioplasmic body, the visible physical body is healed or gradually healed.

The basic techniques used in pranic healing are as follows:

• Sensitizing the hands

• Scanning
    major chakras and relevant minor chakras
    vital organs
    spine

• Cleansing or Sweeping
    General sweeping
    Localized sweeping

- Energizing with Prana
    Drawing in and projecting prana
    Redistributing patient's prana by redistributive sweeping.
- Stabilizing the Projected Prana
    Will Technique
    Blue Prana Technique

Energizing with prana involves two simultaneous actions—that of drawing in prana and that of projecting prana. In order to draw in prana you can use either of the following techniques:

Chakral Technique: Prana is drawn in through a chakra and projected out through the hand chakra. This is done merely by concentrating on the chakra with the intention of drawing in prana.

Pranic Breathing: Prana is drawn in through all parts of the body by using breathing techniques.

Invocative Technique: The healer prays for divine healing energy or prana and requests to be used as a healing instrument.

You can also use a combination of the chakral technique, pranic breathing and the invocative technique.

To project prana you will use either the hand chakra or the finger chakras. Energizing can also be done by redistributing the patient's excess prana to the affected part using redistributive sweeping.

In invocative pranic healing, the healer invokes the help of some mighty spiritual beings in cleansing and energizing the patient.

MEDITATION ON THE TWIN HEARTS

Without leaving the house, one may know all there is in heaven and earth. Without peeping from the window, one may see the ways of heaven. Those who go out learn less and less the more they travel. Wherefore does the sage know all without going anywhere, see all without looking, do nothing and yet achieve (the Goal)!

—Lao Tsu
Tao Te Ching

Meditation should be directed toward the realization of oneness with God. Your entire attention should be given to the realization of God, always bearing in mind that the kingdom of God is within you, neither lo here nor lo there, but within you.

—Joel Goldsmith

Illumination Technique

THE ILLUMINATION TECHNIQUE, or Meditation on the Twin Hearts, is a technique to achieve Buddhic consciousness or cosmic consciousness or illumination. It is also a form of service to the world because the world is harmonized to a certain degree by blessing the entire earth with loving kindness.[7]

Meditation on the Twin Hearts is based on the principle that some of the major chakras are entry points or gateways to certain levels or horizons of consciousness. To achieve illumination or Buddhic consciousness, it is necessary to fully activate the crown chakra. The crown chakra, when fully activated, becomes like a cup. To be more exact, the twelve inner petals open and turn upward like a cup to receive spiritual energies which are distributed to other parts of the body. The crowns worn by kings and queens are but poor physical replicas or symbols of the indescribably resplendent crown chakra of a fully-developed person. The fully activated crown chakra is symbolized as the Holy Grail.

The crown chakra can only be fully activated when the heart chakra is first fully activated. The heart chakra is a replica of the crown chakra.

---

[7]If you want to learn to practice meditation on the twin hearts, please visit the Mei Ling Healing Centers, listed in the Resources section at the back of this book.

When you look at the heart chakra, it looks like the inner chakra of the crown chakra, which has twelve golden petals. The heart chakra is the lower correspondence of the crown chakra. The crown chakra is the center of illumination and divine love or oneness with all. To explain what is divine love and illumination to an ordinary person is just like trying to explain what color is to a blind man. The heart chakra is the center of higher emotions. It is the center for compassion, joy, affection, consideration, mercy and other refined emotions. Without developing higher refined emotions, how can one possibly experience divine love?

There are many ways of activating the heart and crown chakras. You can use physical movements, hatha yoga, yogic breathing techniques, mantras or words of power, and visualization techniques. All of these techniques are effective but are not fast enough. One of the most effective and fastest ways to activate these chakras is to do meditation on loving-kindness or to bless the whole earth with loving-kindness. By using the heart chakra and the crown chakra in blessing the earth with loving-kindness, they become channels for spiritual energies; thereby becoming activated in the process. By blessing the earth with loving-kindness, you are doing a form of world service. And by blessing the earth with loving-kindness, you are in turn blessed many times. It is in blessing that you are blessed. It is in giving that you receive. That is the law!

A person with a fully activated crown chakra does not necessarily achieve illumination for he or she has yet to learn how to make use of the crown chakra to achieve illumination. It is just like having a sophisticated computer but not knowing how to operate it. Once the crown chakra has been fully activated, then you have to do meditation on the light, on the mantra *Aum*,[8] and on the gap between the two Aums. Intense concentration should be focused not only on the mantra Aum but especially on the gap between the two Aums. It is by fully and intensely concentrating on the light and the gap between the two Aums that illumination, or samadhi, is achieved!

With most people, their other chakras are quite activated. The basic chakra, sex chakra, and solar plexus chakra are activated in practically all people. With these people, their instincts for self-survival, sex drive and their tendency to react with their lower emotions are very active. With the pervasiveness of modern education and work that requires the use of the mental faculty, the ajna chakra and the throat chakra are developed in

---

[8]*Aum* is a Sanskrit word for the Supreme Being; in Arabic, *Allah*; in Chinese, *Tao*; and in English, *God*.

a lot of people. What is not developed in most people are the heart and crown chakras. Modern education, unfortunately, tends to overemphasize the development of the throat chakra and the ajna chakra or the development of the concrete mind and the abstract mind. The development of the heart has been neglected. Because of this, you may encounter people who are quite intelligent but very abrasive. This type of person has not yet matured emotionally or the heart chakra is quite underdeveloped. Though he or she is intelligent and may be successful, human relationships are very poor, with hardly any friends and no family or a broken family. By using the meditation on the twin hearts, a person becomes harmoniously balanced.

Whether the abstract and concrete mind will be used constructively or destructivelly depends upon the development of the heart. When the solar plexus chakra is overdeveloped and the heart chakra is underdeveloped, or when the lower emotions are active and the higher emotions are underdeveloped, then the mind would probably be used destructively. Without the development of the heart in most people, world peace will be an unattainable dream. This is why the development of the heart should be emphasized in the educational system.

People less than 18 years old should not practice the illumination technique since the body cannot yet withstand too much subtle energy. This may even manifest as physical paralysis in the long run. People with heart ailments should not practice Meditation on the Twin Hearts since it may result in severe pranic heart congestion. It is important that people who intend to practice Meditation on the Twin Hearts regularly should also practice self-purification or character building through daily inner reflection. Meditation on the Twin Hearts not only activates the heart chakra and the crown chakra but also the other chakras. Because of this, both the positive and negative characteristics of the practitioner will be magnified or activated. This can easily be verified by the practitioner himself and through clairvoyant observation.

PROCEDURE

1) Cleansing the etheric body through physical exercise: Do physical exercise for about five minutes. Doing physical exercise has a cleansing and energizing effect on the etheric body. Light grayish matter or used-up prana is expelled from the etheric body when exercising. Physical exercises

have to be done to minimize possible pranic congestion since this meditation generates a lot of subtle energies in the etheric body.

2) Invocation for divine blessing: Invoking the blessing of one's Spiritual Guides is very important. Each spiritual aspirant has spiritual guides, whether he or she is consciously aware of them or not. The invocation is required for one's protection, help and guidance. Without making the invocation, practicing any advanced meditational technique could be dangerous. You can make your own invocation. I usually use this invocation:

> *Father, I humbly invoke Thy divine blessing!*
> *For protection, guidance, help and*
> *illumination!*
> *With thanks and in full faith!*

3) Activating the heart chakra—blessing the entire earth with loving-kindness: Press your front heart chakra with your finger for a few seconds. This is to make concentration on the front heart chakra easier. Concentrate on the front heart chakra and bless the earth with loving-kindness. You may improvise your own blessing with loving-kindness. I usually use this blessing:

Blessing the Earth with Loving-Kindness

> *From the Heart of God,*
> *Let the entire earth be blessed with*
> *loving-kindness.*
> *Let the entire earth be blessed with great joy,*
> *happiness and divine peace.*
> *Let the entire earth be blessed with*
> *understanding, harmony, good will and*
> *will-to-good. So be it!*

> *From the Heart of God,*
> *Let the hearts of all sentient beings be filled*
> *with divine love and kindness.*
> *Let the hearts of all sentient beings be filled*
> *with great joy, happiness and divine peace.*
> *Let the hearts of all sentient beings be filled*
> *with understanding, harmony, good will and*
> *will-to-good. With thanks, so be it!*

For beginners, this blessing is done only once or twice. Do not overdo this blessing at the start. Some may even feel a slight pranic congestion around the heart area. This is because your etheric body is not sufficiently clean. Apply localized sweeping to remove the congestion.

This blessing should not be done mechanically. You should feel and fully appreciate the implications in each phrase. You may also use visualization. When blessing the earth with loving kindness, visualize the aura of the earth as becoming dazzling pink. When blessing the earth with great joy, happiness and peace, visualize people with heavy difficult problems smiling—their hearts filled with joy, faith, hope and peace. Visualize their problems becoming lighter and their faces lightening up. When blessing the earth with harmony, good will and will-to-good, visualize people or nations on the verge of fighting or fighting each other reconciling. Visualize these people putting down their arms and embracing each other. Visualize them being filled with good intentions and filled with the will to carry out this good intention. This blessing can be directed to a nation or nations, a family or a person or a group of persons. Do not direct this blessing on a specific infant or specific children because they might be overwhelmed by the intense energy generated by the meditation.

4) Activating the crown chakra—blessing the earth with loving-kindness: Press the crown with your finger for several seconds to facilitate concentration on the crown chakra and bless the entire earth with loving-kindness. When the crown chakra is fully opened, some of you will feel something blooming on top of the head and some will also feel something pressing on the crown. After the crown chakra has been activated, concentrate simultaneously on the crown chakra and the heart chakra, and bless the earth with loving-kindness several times. This will align the heart chakra and the crown chakra, thereby making the blessing much more potent.

5) To achieve illumination—meditation on the light, on the Aum and the gap between the two Aums: Visualize a grain of dazzling white light on the crown or at the center inside the head, and simultaneously mentally utter the mantra, Aum. Concentrate intensely on the point of light, on the Aum and on the gap between the two Aums. When mentally uttering the mantra Aum, you will notice that the Aums are not continuous and that there is a slight gap between two mantras or between two Aums. Do this meditation for five to ten minutes. When the spiritual aspirant can fully concentrate simultaneously on the point of light and on the gap

between the two Aums, he or she will experience an "inner explosion of light." The entire being will be filled with light! He or she will have the first glimpse of illumination and the first experience of divine ecstasy! To experience Buddhic consciousness or illumination is to experience and understand what Jesus meant when he said: "If thine eye be single, thy whole body shall be full of light." (Luke 11:34). "For behold, the kingdom of heaven is within you." (Luke 17:21).

For some people, it may take years before they experience an initial glimpse of illumination or Buddhic consciousness. Others may take months while others may take weeks. For the very few, they achieve initial expansion of consciousness on the first try. This is usually done with the help from an elder or a facilitator.

When doing this meditation, the aspirant should be neutral. He or she should not be obsessed with results or filled with too many expectations. Otherwise, he or she will be actually meditating on the expectations or the expected results rather than on the point of light, the Aum and the gap between the two Aums.

6) Releasing excess energy: After the end of the meditation, the excess energy should be released by blessing the earth with Light, Love and Peace. Otherwise, the etheric body will become congested and the visible body will deteriorate in the long run because of too much energy. Other esoteric schools release the excess energy by visualizing the chakras projecting out the excess energy and the chakras becoming smaller and dimmer, but this approach does not put the excess energy into constructive use.

7) Giving thanks: After the end of the meditation, always give thanks to your spiritual guides for the divine blessing.

8) Strengthening the visible physical body through massage and more physical exercises: After the end of the meditation, massage your body and do physical exercise for about five minutes. The purpose is to further cleanse and strengthen the visible body since more used-up prana is expelled out of the body. This facilitates the assimilation of the pranic and spiritual energies, thereby enhancing the beauty and health of the practitioner. Massaging and exercising after this meditation also reduces the possibility of pranic congestion or energy getting in certain parts of the body which may lead to illness. You can also gradually cure yourself of some ailments by doing exercises after doing the Meditation on the Twin Hearts. It is very important to exercise after the meditation; otherwise,

the visible physical body will inevitably be weakened. Although the etheric body will become very bright and strong, the visible physical body will become weak because it will not be able to withstand the leftover energy generated by the meditation in the long run. You have to experience it yourself to fully appreciate what I am saying.

Some of you have the tendency not to do physical exercises after this meditation but to continue savouring the blissful state. This tendency should be overcome, otherwise your physical health will deteriorate in the long run.

Sometimes when a spiritual aspirant meditates, he or she may experience unusual physical movements for a limited period of time. This is quite normal since the etheric channels are being cleansed.

The instructions may seem quite long but the meditation is short, simple and very effective! It requires only ten to fifteen minutes excluding the time required for the physical exercises.

There are many degrees of illumination. The art of "intuiting" or "direct synthetic knowing" requires constant practice (meditation) for a long duration of time. To be more exact, it requires many incarnations to develop facility in the use of this Buddhic faculty.

Blessing the earth with loving-kindness can be done in group as a form of world service. When done in a group for this purpose, first bless the earth with loving-kindness through the heart chakra, then through the crown chakra, then through both the crown chakra and the heart chakra. Release the excess energy after the end of the meditation. The other parts of the meditation are omitted. The blessing can be directed, not only to the entire earth, but also to a specific nation or group of nations. The potency of the blessing is increased many times when done in group. For example, when the blessing is done by a group of seven, the effect or potency is equal to more than one hundred people doing it separately.

Just as pranic healing can miraculously cure simple and severe ailments, the Meditation on Twin Hearts, when practiced by a large number of people can also miraculously heal the entire earth. This message is directed to readers with sufficient maturity and the will-to-good.

• • •

MEDITATION ON THE TWIN HEARTS

1) Clean the etheric body, do physical exercise for about five minutes.

2) Invoke for divine blessing.

3) Activate the heart chakra, concentrate on it, and bless the entire earth with loving-kindness.

4) Activate the crown chakra, concentrate on it, and bless the entire earth with loving-kindness. Then bless the earth with loving-kindness simultaneously through the crown chakra and the heart chakra.

5) To achieve illumination, concentrate on the point of light, on the Aum, and on the gap between the two Aums.

6) To release excess energy, bless the earth with light, love and peace.

7) Give thanks.

8) To strengthen the visible physical body; massage face and body, and do physical exercise for about five minutes.

Meditation on the Twin Hearts is a very powerful tool in bringing about world peace; therefore, this meditational technique should be disseminated. Permission is granted to all interested persons to reprint, recopy, and reproduce the Meditation on the Twin Hearts with proper acknowledgment to both author and publisher.

THE FUTURE OF PRANIC HEALING

Now, my suspicion is that the universe is not only queerer than we suppose, but queerer than we can suppose.

—J.B.S. Haldane,
a British biologist

To each generation is given the part of conserving the essential features of the old and beloved form, but also of wisely expanding and enriching it. Each cycle must add the gain of further research and scientific endeavour, and subtract that which is worn out and of no value.

—by Alice Bailey
Initiation, Human and Solar

Seed Ideas

THE IDEAS CONTAINED HERE are in seed form; therefore, they will require considerable nurturing to fully develop them. They are given as guides and hints to new research areas.

NUTRITION AND PRANA

Science has studied nutrition from the chemical viewpoint: proteins, carbohydrates, sugars, minerals, fats, and vitamins. So far, science is not aware of the existence of prana, and has not studied nutrition from the pranic viewpoint—the quantity and types of color prana contained in foods, and how prana affects the human body.

Preserved food contains more or less the same amount of proteins, carbohydrates, and other chemicals compared to fresh food but fresh food is definitely more nutritious than preserved food because it contains more prana than preserved ones. The same principle also applies to synthetic and natural vitamins. Natural vitamins are more effective or potent than synthetic vitamins because the natural ones contain more prana. Overcooking food not only destroys some of its chemical nutrients but also releases a lot of its prana due to the prolonged heating. In other words, overcooked food contains considerably less prana than food that is not overcooked.

To be healthy, it is necessary to have a balanced diet. The idea of a balanced diet should include not only proper chemical or nutritive mix requirements of the body but also the proper mix of color pranas required to keep the body healthy. To achieve a balanced pranic diet, it is advisable to prepare dishes having many colors. By noting the color of the food, it is possible to deduce the predominating color prana. For example, green vegetables obviously contain a lot of green prana while carrots contain a lot of orange prana. But this approach is not always applicable; for instance, red tomatoes contain a lot of greenish-yellow prana and very little red prana, and watermelons which have smooth green skin and red pulp contain a lot of green prana and hardly any red prana.

The approach of Western medicine is very different from Chinese medicine or Ayurvedic (Indian) medicine. With Western medicine, the approach is material or chemical. With Chinese or Ayurvedic medicine, the approach is more subtle. What is emphasized in Chinese and Ayurvedic medicine is pranic energy and maintaining pranic harmony within the body. Chinese medicine has developed this approach to a very sophisticated degree using herbal medicine and acupuncture.

It is commonly known that hemorrhoids tend to worsen by eating hot spicy foods. Why is this so? The answer is quite simple. Since hemorrhoids manifest as pranic congestion of red prana on the anus area, eating hot spicy foods, which contain a lot of red prana, would definitely aggravate the ailment.

People who are susceptible to constipation may improve their condition by regularly eating papaya. Papaya contains a lot of orange prana which stimulates regular bowel movements.

According to some writers, violet grapes have miraculous healing effects. They claim that there are some cancer patients and other patients with severe ailments that have been cured through the grape diet. The skin of violet grapes contains predominantly violet prana and its pulp contains predominantly greenish-yellow prana. Violet prana is a powerful kind of prana, having the properties of all the other color pranas. It has disinfecting and detoxifying effects, and is also used to destroy cancerous cells. Violet prana and yellowish-green prana have regenerating effects, and are used to accelerate the repair of damaged organs. More thorough research should be directed toward the study of violet grapes as a possible cure for cancer, damaged internal organs, AIDS, and other severe ailments.

The research should not only focus on the visible physical body but also its effects on the bioplasmic body. Research should also be directed toward the use of combining a violet grape diet and ginseng as a cure for some incurable ailments. The expectations for both researchers and patients should be realistic; they have to take into account the karmic factor, and the severe damage already done to the patient's physical body due to the ailment, and the serious side effects of potent drugs that were used.

GINSENG

Experiments have been done on the effects of Chinese and Korean red ginseng on the etheric body. The dosage used ranges from one-half a gram to five grams per intake. The subjects' ages ranged from 14 to 55 years old.

It was clairvoyantly observed that the effects of ginseng powder start to manifest almost immediately. Flashes of light were seen coming from the inner and health auras. The inner aura increased from five to about ten inches in thickness. The health aura became brighter and expanded from two to three feet. The outer aura also expanded. Light grayish matter was being expelled. The chakras became brighter, bigger and more active. The major chakras increased from three-and-a-half inches to about five inches. The "synthetic ki" located at the secondary navel chakras increased from one inch to about three inches in diameter. The "synthetic ki" became denser. Although the pranic energy level of the subjects was very high, they were relaxed and not restless. This is similar to a person meditating. Though a lot of energy is generated when meditating, the meditator is still relaxed and at peace. The subjects are not usually aware or do not physically feel the subtle improvements unless they are either sensitive or weak.

The degree of the effects of the ginseng depends on the dosage, the supplier of the ginseng (different suppliers produce ginseng of different brightness or potency), and the body of the subject. The effects of one-half a gram of ginseng will last for about ten to sixteen hours. Within that period of time the effects of the ginseng gradually diminish. Because of this, it is better if one-half a gram of ginseng is taken twice a day to maintain one's health. People who are ill should preferably take a higher dosage.

Ginseng, when clairvoyantly seen, is very bright compared to other food and medicines. The core (inmost) aura of a fifty gram red ginseng powder is very dense (looks almost like "liquid" gold) and is six to twelve inches in radius. The next layer of the aura is three to six feet in radius. The outer aura is nine to twelve feet in radius. Ginseng contains a lot of prana (vital energy) and also a lot of "synthetic ki." The great increase of "synthetic ki" in the secondary navel chakra is due to the activated major chakras which produce more "synthetic ki" and also due to the "synthetic ki" contained in the ginseng itself.

Ginseng has a cleansing effect since grayish matter is being expelled. It is better to exercise immediately after taking ginseng to facilitate the expelling of used-up prana and to facilitate the assimilation of fresh pranic energy. Ginseng is also activating and energizing since the etheric body and its major chakras become brighter, bigger and denser. Therefore, the organs controlled and energized by the major chakras are correspondingly cleansed, activated and energized.

With these findings, it becomes clear why ginseng is highly regarded by the Chinese and Koreans. Many Chinese and Koreans take ginseng regularly to improve and maintain their good health. In Chinese medicine, ginseng in combination with herbs having healing effects on a specific organ, or which carry or direct the chi energy to a specific organ, are prescribed for many types of ailments. Ginseng combined with other herbs is considered as a practically cure all medicine.

To increase the pranic energy level of the healer and to improve his or her healing skill, it is advisable (but not necessary) to take one gram of ginseng before and after healing a large number of patients. It is also advantageous for patients who are very weak to take one to two grams of ginseng before being treated by the healer.

CLASSIFYING DRUGS BY COLOR PRANA

A person who has just embarked on the study and research of the different properties and effects of herbs and drugs is sometimes overwhelmed by the huge body of information available. A different approach to classification of herbs and drugs is suggested by using the properties of color prana. A chart can be made to give an overall view. The vertical side of the chart will contain a list of color pranas, mixed color pranas, and their corresponding properties. The horizontal side of the chart will contain first the whole body followed by its different specific parts. Herbs or drugs are then cataloged in the chart. A diuretic drug (promotes secretion of urine) is cataloged under orange prana or yellowish-green prana—expelling property, and the kidneys. Analgesic or pain killer is cataloged under blue prana—soothing effect, and the body. The herb or groups of herbs with dissolving effects on blood clots or clogs is cataloged under green prana—breaking down or dissolving effects, and the whole body. The herb or group of herbs with decongesting or cleansing effects on the heart is cataloged under green prana—dissolving and decongesting effects, and the heart. The herb or group of herbs which accelerate the repair process of the heart is cataloged under violet prana, and green-yellow prana—regenerating effects, and the heart. To fill the chart would require considerable amount of time and energy, and the concerted efforts of many experienced herbalists and pharmacists.

HYGIENE AND DISEASED BIOPLASMIC MATTER

The study of hygiene should include not only germs and dirt but also diseased bioplasmic matter or diseased energy. This diseased bioplasmic matter or diseased energy can be transmitted to another person. In the earlier chapters, you learned about sweeping in order to remove diseased etheric matter or diseased energy. Some of you may have experienced pain or discomfort on the hands when applying sweeping and energizing. A healer who does not throw away the diseased energy and does not wash his or her hands after treatment may experience the symptoms or ailments of the patients. This will severely affect the health of the healer in the long run.

You can experiment by regularly throwing the diseased energy of your patients to a plant. The plant will definitely weaken and gradually die if the experiment is continued for a prolonged period of time.

A hospital room that is relatively free of germs but has been occupied by many severely sick patients may in the long run become etherically very dirty. In such a case, the room is considered "unlucky" by the medical personnel working in the hospital. They are aware that such a room tends to have a higher mortality rate but they do not understand why. It is advisable to etherically clean hospital rooms at regular intervals, especially those rooms occupied by severely sick patients and those who are suffering from lingering, depressive, and very painful ailments.

There are several ways of etherically cleaning a room. The first method is to open the curtains and windows to let sunlight and fresh air in for several days or even weeks. This is exactly what some shamans or American Indian healers are doing. They extract diseased energy from the patient and deposit the diseased energy in a container filled with tobacco and water (bioplasmic waste disposal unit). The container is then exposed to sunlight and wind in order to gradually disintegrate the diseased energy.

The second method is to expose the room to orange and green lights for several hours. Green light, and orange light have disintegrating and expelling effects on the diseased bioplasmic matter.

The third method is to use religious rituals. Incense, salt water and prayer are used. Different types of incense and perfumes have different effects on bioplasmic matter. Some incense (like sandalwood) has cleansing effects while others have cementing or solidifying effects. Hence, you cannot just use any type of incense for cleansing.

Diseased energy can also transmit psychological ailments. When a patient talks about psychological problems, pent-up negative emotional energy in the form of diseased bioplasmic matter is released by the patient and is usually absorbed by the psychotherapist, especially if the psychotherapist is quite open, understanding and compassionate. The release of negative emotional energy is clairvoyantly seen as a brightening up of the patient's auras due to the release of grayish energy of different colors.

The unconscious absorption of this negative energy by the psychotherapist produces immediate and long run problems. The immediate problem may manifest as a family problem, since the psychotherapist may try to unconsciously release the negative energy or take it out on immediate members of the family. Under normal circumstances, the body's defense system can expel the negative energy and recover just through a good night's sleep. But since this is done regularly, the negative emotional energy in the form of diseased bioplasmic matter accumulates and inevitably manifests as chakral imbalances. These chakral imbalances may manifest as psychological problems or symptoms similar to the patient's. It may manifest physically as a low energy level or burn-out, heart problems, chest pains, rapid aging, or other physical ailments.

And how can healers protect themselves from negative emotional energy? There are already several books written about this. See suggested reading in esoteric practices. I may also seriously consider writing a book on pranic psychotherapy in the near future.

ROTATION OF THE CHAKRAS

In what direction does a chakra rotate? Some students think it rotates counterclockwise; some think it rotates clockwise. Both are partially correct and partially wrong. A chakra is rapidly rotating alternately clockwise and counterclockwise. Clockwise motion draws in pranic energy to the chakra, while counterclockwise motion projects or draws out pranic energy from the chakra. Clockwise motion of the chakra is absorbing, while counterclockwise motion of the chakra is projecting or expelling. When a healer draws in pranic energy through a chakra, the chakra is predominantly rotating clockwise, and to a much lesser degree, rotating counterclockwise. When a healer projects pranic energy through a chakra, it is predominantly rotating counterclockwise, and to a much lesser degree, rotating clockwise. Under normal conditions, a chakra is rotating clockwise and counterclockwise in equal proportion. So the amount of pranic energy coming in and going out is about the same.

When energizing, the hand chakra is predominantly rotating counterclockwise and to a lesser degree clockwise (drawing in). This is why the energizing hand also absorbs diseased energy and has to be flicked regularly to throw away the diseased energy. It is better to clean before energizing, not only to reduce the possibility of radical reaction, but also to minimize the quantity of diseased energy that will be absorbed by the healer when energizing. This is why I do not recommend that healers energize with the use of their eyes or with a major chakra because the eyes are very delicate and difficult to clean and a major chakra controls a vital organ or several organs. There is the possibility that the corresponding organ or organs would fully absorb the diseased energy which would be harmful to the healers.

Under normal conditions, a chakra is drawing in and projecting pranic energy alternately at a rapid rate. The amount of pranic energy drawn in and projected is more or less equal. The chakra rotates clockwise at 180 degrees and counterclockwise at 180 degrees in the opposite direction alternately at a rapid rate. When the hand chakra predominantly projects, the counterclockwise motion is 360 degrees and the clockwise motion is only 180 degrees. When the hand chakra rotates counterclockwise, it projects pranic energy and stops for a split second, then rotates in clockwise motion and draws in pranic energy and stops for a split second. The entire process is repeated. The pranic energy projected is not continuous, nor is the pranic energy drawn in continuous. It only appears as continuous because the chakra is moving rapidly and alternately clockwise and counterclockwise, thereby giving an appearance of continuous projection of pranic energy or continuous drawing in of pranic energy. The difference in the intensity of pranic energy projected depends upon the rate of rotation of the chakras. The faster it rotates, the more intense is the projected pranic energy and the slower it rotates, the less intense is the pranic energy projected. When a hand chakra is predominantly absorbing it makes a 360 degree clockwise rotation and a 180 degree counterclockwise rotation and vice versa when it is predominantly projecting pranic energy. The intensity of pranic energy projected or absorbed does not involve changes in the pattern of rotation of the chakra, but is dependent upon the rate of rotation of the chakra. The faster it rotates, the more intense is the projected or absorbed prana.

In India, there are yogis who heal by placing one hand near the affected part, then moving it in circular motion. If the yogi wants to clean or decongest an affected part, he applies localized sweeping by moving his hand several times in a counterclockwise motion with the intention of increasing the chakra's counterclockwise motion, thereby facilitating the removal of diseased energy. He then flicks his hand to throw away the diseased energy. This process is continued until the affected chakra becomes substantially clean. If the yogi wants to energize an affected chakra, he projects pranic energy and simultaneously moves his hand clockwise with the intention of making the affected chakra draw in more pranic energy by increasing the chakra's clockwise motion. Clockwise motion is drawing in while counterclockwise motion is drawing out or decongesting. The technique is simple and easy to apply.

The appearance of the chakra is dependent upon its speed of rotation. Under normal conditions, the rapid clockwise and counterclockwise rotations produce an optical effect making the chakra look like a lotus flower with many pointed petals. The pointed petals are optically produced by the combined motion of pranic energy moving clockwise and counterclockwise. This is why in ancient Tibetan, Chinese and Sanskrit books on yoga, the chakras are usually presented as lotus flowers with many pointed petals. When a chakra is deliberately slowed down, the actual shape and number of petals can be clearly seen. The shape of the petals of a chakra is round. This is why the petals of the chakras described by Leadbeater are round, not pointed. When the chakra is moving very rapidly, the chakra bulges out or becomes quite thick. When it is rotating at an extremely rapid rate, the chakra appears as a dazzling point of light. When a spiritual aspirant is meditating, spiritual and pranic energies are attracted to the head area. This is why advanced yogis or saints are clairvoyantly seen with dazzling or blinding light on the head area (a spiritual halo).

GEOMETRIC PRANIC GENERATORS

A four-sided pyramid, a three-sided pyramid, and a cone generate or focus pranic energy or vitality globules within itself. More air vitality globules are contained within these geometric figures than in the air, hence, they are called pranic generators. The pranic energy or air vitality globules in these geometric figures is as dense, if not denser, than the ground prana or vitality globules. Recuperating inside a geometric pranic generator is similar to resting and recuperating on the ground in order to absorb ground pranic energy. Better results can be obtained by cleansing the body with the application of general and localized sweeping. See figure 42.

Experiments can be done by wearing a cone headgear on top of the crown to increase one's learning capacity, to think faster and more clearly, and to make better decisions. This is probably why ancient magicians or wise men are sometimes depicted with cone-shaped headgear.

Healing or treating patients inside a geometric pranic generator is a lot easier. Since the healing space or area is filled with dense pranic energy, drawing in pranic energy and projecting pranic energy can be done faster and with greater ease. Very often using a three-dimensional geometric pranic generator is not possible. A two-dimensional geometric pranic gen-

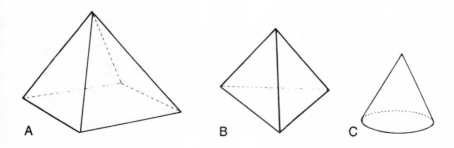

Figure 42. Three-dimensional pranic generators: (A) four-sided pyramid; (B) three-sided pyramid; and (C) cone.

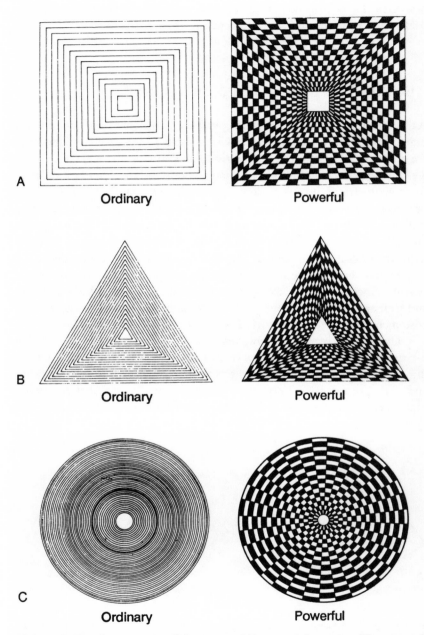

A   Ordinary   Powerful

B   Ordinary   Powerful

C   Ordinary   Powerful

Figure 43. Pranic generators of three types: (A) concentric square; (B) concentric triangle; and (C) concentric circle.

erator can be used. Concentric squares, triangles, and circles are two-dimensional geometric pranic generators. See figure 43. There are many variations of these two-dimensional pranic generators. They are less potent than the three-dimensional ones but are still considerably potent and useful. The wall or floor where the pranic treatment will be given can be designed with a two-dimensional geometric pranic generator. It is better to use only one design, not several combined designs, because it will cause confusion in the etheric bodies of people within the geometric pranic generator. It is better to use the square or the triangle designs rather than the circle design, since some patients may not be able to withstand the type of pranic energy generated by the cone or the concentric circle design.

PRANIC LASER THERAPY

In healing with the use of color lights (or chromotherapy), some healers have the wrong concept that it is color alone that heals. Unless this concept is corrected, progress in this field will remain slow. It is not color that heals, but the vitality globules or pranic energy that has been transformed by the color light to a specific color prana that heals. Obviously, the density or the quantity of pranic energy (vitality globules) in the healing room is a very critical factor. If the healing room contains more pranic energy, then the pranic treatment will be more effective and vice versa. This is why it is advisable to use a geometric pranic generator to increase the quantity of air prana in the healing room.

Another important factor is the degree of permanency or stability of the transformed color pranic energy. This is dependent upon the distance between the treated part and the source of color light. If the distance is too short, the transformed color prana will revert back to white prana. Although the treatment will still be effective, it will not be as effective as when the transformed color pranic energy remains as is. As discussed in the earlier chapter, color prana is faster and more effective than white prana when used correctly.

The potency of pranic energy is affected by its velocity and rate of vibration. The velocity of the pranic energy is affected by the distance. The further the distance between the treated part and the source of color light, the faster is the velocity of the vitality globules. If the distance is too short, the velocity is not fast enough; therefore the potency of pranic energy is not strong enough. If the distance is too far, the velocity of the vitality globules will also be very fast. This may result in some damaging effects.

The use of soft laser light in pranic therapy (laser pranic therapy) is a more advanced form of pranic chromotherapy. The effect of pranic laser therapy is very fast, comparable to pranic treatment done by an advanced pranic healer. Mei Ling prophesied that a few decades from now pranic laser therapy will be widely used. The following guidelines are suggested by my teacher, Mei Ling:

1) The substance used in generating laser light should have a carbon content ranging from fifty to eighty percent. Within this range, the pranic laser treatment is quite effective. Below this range, it is not so effective. And beyond this range, the treatment will have destructive effects. It may be necessary to synthetically produce this substance.

2) The distance between the part to be treated and the source of laser light should range from one to five feet. The distance affects the degree of permanency of the transformed prana and the potency of the projected pranic energy (velocity of the projected prana). If it is too far, the velocity of the projected vitality globules would be too fast and would have a damaging effect.

3) The power or wattage should preferably range from fifteen to twenty-five watts. If the wattage is too low, it will not be very effective. If it is too high, it will be destructive.

4) In general, exposure time should range from one to seven seconds. If the exposure time is too short, the projected pranic energy will not be sufficient. If the exposure time is too long, there will be an overdose.

The healing room should preferably have a geometric pranic generator. This increases the density or the amount of air vitality globules in the healing room. The patient should be scanned before and after treatment. General and localized sweeping should be applied before energizing. Further localized sweeping may be required after energizing. While energizing, the projected pranic energy should be directed to the affected organ and should be stabilized.

An experiment can be done on the rapid healing of fresh wounds with the simultaneous use of soft red laser light and soft orange laser light. The given guidelines should not be accepted blindly, but should be studied thoroughly and its validity tested through thorough experiments.

Knowledge is neither good nor bad. It is how we make use of it that makes it good or bad. Hence, the development of the heart should be emphasized, especially, among scientists, businessmen, and politicians.

> . . . that we must not believe in a thing said merely because it is said; nor traditions because they have been handed down from antiquity; nor rumors, as such; nor writings by sages, because sages wrote them; nor fancies that we may suspect to have been inspired in us by a Deva [that is, in presumed spiritual inspiration]; nor from inferences drawn from some haphazard assumption we may have made; nor because of what seems an analogical necessity; nor on the mere authority of our teachers or masters. But we are to believe when the writing, doctrine, or saying is corroborated by our own reason and consciousness. "For this," says he in concluding, "I taught you not to believe merely because you have heard, but when you believed of your consciousness, then to act accordingly and abundantly."[9]

---

[9]Lord Buddha as quoted in Helena Blavatsky, *Secret Doctrine*, Vol. III (Wheaton, IL: Theosophical Publishing House, 1980), p. 401.

APPENDICES

Testimonials

DATE: December 23, 1986
NAME: Mrs. Pia A. Victoria
AGE: 59
OCCUPATION: Housewife

CASE: *Glaucoma and Chest Pains*

Q: What was your health condition before?
Pia: I had glaucoma and frequent chest pains which were troubling me.

Q: Did you consult a medical doctor or a specialist before seeing a pranic healer?
Pia: Yes, and the doctor diagnosed my eye ailment as glaucoma. With regard to my chest pains, I had a general medical examination and there was no indication that I had a heart ailment or one developing. However, during the checkup, I did not have an electrocardiogram examination.

In the beginning, I was skeptical about pranic healing, so for a try, I had my eyes treated first.

Q: What did you feel when pranic healing was applied on your eyes?

Pia: I felt some relief or a soothing effect, then later on I could see a little brighter. The effects were not immediate since I felt the relief thirty minutes or an hour later.

Q: How often do you get this pranic treatment?

Pia: It depends whether I was busy or not. It was very irregular. Before, I used to have it once a week, then later on once in three weeks.

Q: Is your eye ailment getting better or is there an improvement after pranic treatment?

Pia: My right eye is okay now but there seems to be no improvement with my left eye. Everytime I get tense and excited, the condition of my left eye worsens.

My frequent chest pains were also cured after pranic treatments because I do not experience them anymore or if ever they recur, it's very, very seldom. Previously, I used to have them very often and since there was no change in my lifestyle, there was no medication taken or applied except for several pranic treatments, then I am certain that this could have been the effect of such treatments.

DATE:	December 26, 1986
NAME:	Allan C. Cañete
AGE:	24
OCCUPATION:	Student
CASE:	*One Day Old Wound*

Q: Describe the condition of your wound before the pranic treatment.

Allan: I had stepped on a sharp seashell. The width of the wound on the sole of my left foot was about ¼ inch. There was a little bleeding but it was very painful which was caused by a small seashell particle left inside the wound. I had tried all the means within my reach to remove it but to no avail. No medicine was administered before, during, and after the application of pranic healing.

Q: How old was the wound when it was treated with pranic healing and was it infected before the treatment?

Allan: The wound was one day old and I could no longer use my left foot. It was not infected but symptoms showed that it may lead to infection.

Q: Who administered pranic healing on your wound? What happened during and after the treatments?

Allan: I received two successive pranic treatments. The first one was given by Sandra Torrijos (author's student in pranic healing). Actually, the process was just an experiment on rapid healing which was suggested by the author to Sandra. It took Sandra approximately two hours to relieve me of the pain, to close and to partially heal the wound. But since the seashell particle was still inside it, I still had slight difficulty in walking.

The second treatment was administered by the author and *it only took him one-and-a-half hours to rapidly and completely heal my wound right before my eyes!* During the process (both the first and the second treatments), I could feel a tickling, tingling sensation even if there was no skin contact because the distance between the healer's hand and my wound was about one centimeter apart. After the second treatment, I could feel very little pain and my left foot could be used for walking again even if the seashell particle was still inside the healed wound. After two days I removed the seashell with my fingernails.

Q: What can you say about the pranic treatments administered on your wound?

Allan: The technique is very strange but the result is amazing and very effective. In the ordinary method of treating a wound, it would take several days to have it healed, but with pranic healing, it took only three-and-a-half hours to heal the wound right before my eyes.

DATE:	December 26, 1986
NAME:	Romualdo Cañete
AGE:	49
OCCUPATION:	Musician

CASE:	*Cardiac Injury*

Q: What was your health condition before and when was that?

Romualdo: There was severe pain in the area around my right chest and I felt as if half my body was being paralyzed. My blood pressure was higher than normal, the beating of my heart was faster than normal, and I perspired abnormally. The area around my hips was aching, too. I was very sick then, which happened last September 1985.

Q: Did you consult a medical doctor, or a specialist about your illness before seeing a pranic healer? If so, why did you see a pranic healer?

Romualdo: Yes, I first consulted a cardiologist, then a pranic healer for treatment because my son, Allan, recommended the healer. Besides I wanted to recover immediately from my illness. Since I also wanted to compare both methods, I was seeing my cardiologist and my pranic healer alternately. But I did not inform my cardiologist that I was having pranic treatments, too.

Q: What was the diagnosis of your cardiologist and the pranic healer? Can you give some comments about the two methods of treatment administered to you?

Romualdo: The cardiologist and the pranic healer had almost the same findings. The former told me that I have a cardiac injury and the latter told me there is something wrong with my heart because of some cholesterol deposits in it. However, the cardiologist did not discover the pain around my hips that had been troubling me for quite some time, but the healer did.

After an electrocardiogram examination, the cardiologist prescribed various kinds of medicines and cautioned me to take them religiously to prevent a future fatal heart attack. He also told me to go on a strict diet.

During my last visit to the cardiologist, he made a remark on my rapid recovery as compared with other patients. Usually those who have my illness were hospitalized and had not yet recovered by that time. I was also surprised with the X-ray result conducted by my company. I was certain of a heart damage indication but it only indicated a shadow and that *I am fit to work.* The said X-ray was taken around the first week of December, 1986, and this was my first one since the time I had recovered from my illness. I remembered what the pranic healer said on my last visit, "You are already cured!"

Q: How many healing sessions were administered to you by the pranic healer?

Romualdo: I cannot remember the number of pranic treatments, but I am sure that I had been seeing the healer for treatment for less than a month, maybe four to five times.

Q: Who treated you? What did you feel during and after the pranic treatments?

Romualdo: It was Mike Nator (healer friend of the author) who treated me first while the succeeding treatments were done by the author. After the first two treatments, I felt the relief from all the physical discomforts I had before, because the feeling of numbness was gone and the pain was lessened. I did not feel anything during the succeeding treatments.

Presently, I am doing things that I could not perform before, like climbing the overpass, running without panting, and carrying or pushing heavy things. The pain around my hips vanished but it comes back whenever I eat salty and fatty food.

After my rapid recovery, I have not gone back to my cardiologist nor to my pranic healer. I am still taking the prescribed medicine but very irregularly.

Q: What do you think is the role of pranic healing in the rapid recovery of your ailment?

Romualdo: I think pranic healing played a great role on my fast recovery. Just like the comment of my cardiologist about my rapid recovery from cardiac injury. Ordinarily, patients with cardiac injury should be hospitalized. And it would take them considerable time to recover from such illness. In my case, I was not hospitalized and it took me less than a month to recover plus the fact that there was no indication of heart damage or injury that appeared in my X-ray report.

DATE:	January 28, 1987
NAME:	Mrs. Luz Jubay
AGE:	24
OCCUPATION:	Housewife
CASE:	*Prevented Possible Miscarriage*

Q: What was ailing you before you consulted a pranic healer?

Luz: I was two months pregnant (my first one), and the area around my abdomen was aching acutely. I was also bleeding.

Q: Did you consult a medical doctor first before pranic treatment?

Luz: Yes, and the doctor informed me of a possible miscarriage. He prescribed a medication to prevent it but wasn't certain of its potency. I was also advised to take complete rest and to avoid too much physical exertion. I took several doses of the prescribed medication but the pain around my abdomen persisted although the bleeding had stopped.

Q: Did you see a pranic healer immediately after the medical treatment? What happened during and after the pranic treatment?

Luz: I went to see a pranic healer the day after I had my medical treatment. I did not feel anything during the pranic treatment but the pain around my abdomen disappeared. It has not recurred and now I am seven months pregnant. A very mild pain recurs occasionally if I take long walks and also when I carry or push heavy things. This is probably normal for pregnant women.

Q: How many times were you given pranic treatments, and what was the duration for each treatment?

Luz: Only once. And it took the healer about five minutes to administer it.

Q: Who treated you?

Luz: The author.

Q: What do you think is the role of pranic healing in the prevention of your miscarriage?

Luz: I think it helped and contributed in a way for the prevention of my possible miscarriage. I just cannot fully determine its degree of effectiveness since I had taken three possible alternative treatments like the prescribed medication, complete rest, and pranic healing.

DATE:	January 10, 1987
NAME:	Teofilo P. Velasco
AGE:	68
OCCUPATION:	Lawyer
CASE:	*Heart Ailment and Hardened Muscles*

Q: What was your health condition before?

Teofilo: Before both my hands were shaking very obviously; my back, knees, and all down below were aching; my legs were weak and the muscles were hardened; I had frequent and continuous chest pains. It started ten years ago even when I was on medication prescribed by a doctor.

Since I had shaky hands, somebody had to assist me when I ate my meals because I could not bring the food and drink to my mouth without spilling. I could not walk faster the way I used to do and could not even walk immediately after getting up from bed.

Q: What is your present health condition?

Teofilo: I have improved a lot after the author treated me and prayed over me several times. I can eat alone now because my hands no longer shake. The muscles of my legs are all right because I can now walk faster. Maybe this is the effect of the energized oil given to me by the author because since I started using it last January 1, 1987, I felt that the muscles of my legs and feet were loosened and softened. The pain in my back has disappeared but sometimes it recurs when I exert too much effort. I am also getting well from my frequent and continuous chest pains because I only experience it when I am very tired, excited or emotionally upset.

Q: Are you still on medication?

Teofilo: Yes, but very irregularly. However, there is one medication that had been prescribed by my doctor that I was advised to take everyday till I die. But I feel and believe that it is not necessary to do so. That's why I am not taking the medication anymore.

Q: What did you feel when you were being healed?

Teofilo: I felt my body becoming lighter, and my muscles being activated. Also, something was being cleansed from my body by some mysterious force. This makes me feel better.

Q: How many pranic healing sessions were administered to you?

Teofilo: I cannot really remember anymore. There were irregular healing sessions because I would just have the treatments whenever I visit the author. Usually, twice a week.

DATE:	January 15, 1987
NAME:	Mrs. Merlita delos Santos
OCCUPATION:	Beautician
CASE:	*Urinary Ailment*

Q: What was the illness of your son before?

Merly: He had a kidney ailment and the symptoms during the first attack were severe. He had high blood pressure, high fever, generalized edema, difficulty in breathing and discharging urine from the body, and pain in the area around his urinary bladder and ureters. His urine was reddish in color. He got tired very easily. (Alvin was five years old then and in prep school. His studies were interrupted because of his ailment.)

There was a recurrence when he was six. There was an interval of approximately six months from the first attack. His studies then were also interrupted. The symptoms during the second attack were not as severe as compared to the first one. He had pain in the area around the urinary bladder and ureters, and had difficulty urinating and the color of his urine was deep yellow.

Q: Did you bring him to a doctor or to a medical specialist for treatment? What was the development?

Merly: I brought him to a medical (kidney) specialist for treatment. The medication given for the first and second attacks were the same and it greatly relieved him of most discomforts except for the pain around the urinary bladder and ureters. He was advised to avoid too much physical exertion—that means no playing, which is a torment for a child like my son.

Q: Was there a recurrence after the second attack?

Merly: Yes. In the third attack, he experienced a piercing pain in the area around the urinary bladder and ureters. He still had difficulty discharging urine and its color was yellow-orange. I did not let him take any pills or medication. And instead of bringing him to a medical specialist, we went to see a pranic healer for treatment. The pranic healer advised me not to include salty foods in Alvin's diet. (Alvin was seven years old then and in first grade.)

Q: How many times was he treated with pranic healing?

Merly: Three times within two weeks.

Q: After all those pranic treatments, what was the health condition of your son?

Merly: There was a dramatic change and improvement in his condition because his ailment up to now has not recurred. Before, he got tired very easily. But now he plays like other children. The difficulty in passing urine and the piercing pain he felt has completely disappeared. His studies have not been interrupted so far.

DATE: February 23, 1987
NAME: Michael C. Chua
AGE: 26

CASE: *Pancreatitis*

Q: What was the nature of your ailment? What were the symptoms?

Michael: I was vomiting several times. My body was cold and I was chilling and shivering. I felt an intense pain in my solar plexus area. The condition of my body was terrible. The doctor diagnosed it as acute pancreatitis.

Q: Were you hospitalized? Were you treated by a medical specialist? Did you have blood tests?

Michael: I was hospitalized and was treated by a medical specialist. I went through several blood tests and ultrasound examination.

Q: What happened during and after pranic healing?

Michael: I was treated once in the morning, in the afternoon, and in the evening. I did not feel anything during the pranic treatments given to me, but after the last treatment I vomited and after about thirty minutes the pain completely disappeared. My body became normal.

Q: Was there a recurrence?

Michael: There was no recurrence.

Q: What do you think is the role of pranic healing in your recovery?

Michael: I think pranic healing contributed a lot to my rapid recovery.

Resources

MEI LING HEALING CENTERS

30 Kamuning Road
Quezon City
Manila, Philippines

261-A Rodriguez St.
cor. H. Lopez Boulevard
Balut, Tondo
Manila, Philippines

Barangay Hall
San Mateo St.
Makati
Manila, Philippines

ESOTERIC ORGANIZATIONS

These esoteric organizations would be very happy to help and guide spiritual aspirants in their studies and practices. All you have to do is write to them and request a catalog or introductory material. Enclose a self-addressed stamped envelope.

Agni Yoga Society
319 West 107th Street
New York, NY 10025

A.M.O.R.C.
Rosicrucian Order
Rosicrucian Park
San Jose, CA 95191

The Arcane School
113 University Place
11th Floor
New York, NY 10003

Astara
800 W. Arrow Highway
PO Box 5003
Upland, CA 91785

Builders of the Adytum
5105 N. Figueroa Street
Los Angeles, CA 90042

The Rosicrucian Fellowship
PO Box 173
Oceanside, CA 92054

Self-Realization Fellowship
3880 San Rafael Avenue
Los Angeles, CA 90065

Sufi Order
408 Precita Avenue
San Francisco, CA 94110

Theosophical Society
Adyar, Madras 600020
India

Theosophical Society
in the Philippines
1 Iba Street corner of
P. Florentino Street
Quezon City
Manila, Philippines

Recommended Reading

For serious spiritual aspirants, these books are a must for study and practice. They have been arranged in such a way that the aspirant will be guided step by step, thereby avoiding confusion and waste of time and energy. Books are arranged from easy to difficult, and are grouped together according to the nature of the discipline.

ESOTERIC TEACHINGS

Heindel, Max. *The Rosicrucian Cosmo-Conception*. Oceanside, CA: The Rosicrucian Fellowship.

Powell, Arthur E. *The Etheric Double*. Quest Books: Wheaton, IL: Theosophical Publishing House.

———. *The Astral Body*. Wheaton, IL: Theosophical Publishing House.

———. *The Mental Body*. Wheaton, IL: Theosophical Publishing House.

———. *The Causal Body and the Ego*. Quest Books: Wheaton, IL: Theosophical Publishing House.

The Southern Centre of Theosophy. *Devas and Men*. Wheaton, IL: Theosophical Publishing House.

Wood, Ernest. *The Seven Rays*. Quest Books: Wheaton, IL: Theosophical Publishing House.

Baynes, C. F. and R. Wilhelm. *The I Ching or Book of Changes*. Bollingen Series, No. 19. Princeton, NJ: Princeton University Press, 1967.

Krishnamurti. *Education and Significance in Life*. New York: Harper & Row, 1981.

Bailey, Alice A. *Education in the New Age*. New York: Lucis Publishing Company.

———. *From Intellect to Intuition*. New York: Lucis Publishing Company.

———. *Initiation: Human and Solar*. New York: Lucis Publishing Company.

———. *The Rays and Initiations* (Vol. 5). New York: Lucis Publishing Company.

———. *The Externalisation of the Hierarchy*. New York: Lucis Publishing Company.

Hall, Manly P. *Freemasonry of the Ancient Egyptians*. Los Angeles: Philosophical Research Society.

———. *The Lost Keys of Freemasonry*. Richmond, VA: Macoy Publishing, 1981.

———. *The Hidden Life in Freemasonry*. Wheaton, IL: Theosophical Publishing House.

Leadbeater, C. W. *Ancient Mystic Rites* (Orig: *Glimpses of Masonic History*.) Wheaton, IL: Theosophical Publishing House.

ESOTERIC PRACTICES

Yogananda, Paramahansa. *Autobiography of a Yogi*. Los Angeles: Self-Realization Fellowship.

Krishnamurti, J. *At the Feet of the Master*. Wheaton, IL: Theosophical Publishing House.

Slater, Wallace. *Raja Yoga*. Wheaton, IL: Theosophical Publishing House.

Rieker, Hans-Ulrich. *The Yoga of Light*. Lower Lake, CA: Dawn Horse Press.

Motoyama, Hiroshi. *Theories of the Chakra: Bridge to Higher Consciousness*. Quest Books: Wheaton, IL: Theosophical Publishing House.

Kriyananda, Goswami. *The Spiritual Science of Kriya Yoga*. Chicago: Temple of Kriya Yoga.

Brunton, Paul. *The Secret Path*. York Beach, ME: Samuel Weiser.

Vivekananda, Swami. *Raja-Yoga*. New York: Ramakrisna Vivekananda Center.

Hope, Murray. *Practical Techniques of Psychic Self-Defense*. New York: St. Martins; and Wellingborough, England: Aquarian Press.

Mickaharic, Draja. *Spiritual Cleansing: A Handbook of Psychic Protection*. York Beach, ME: Samuel Weiser.

Weed, Joseph J. *Complete Guide to Oracle and Prophesy Methods*. Wellingborough, England: A. Thomas & Company.

Schwartz, Jack. *Voluntary Controls: Exercises for Creative Meditation and for Activating the Potential of the Chakras*. New York: Dutton.

Dael. *The Crystal Book*. Sunol, CA: Crystal Company.

Silbey, Uma. *The Complete Crystal Guidebook*. New York: Bantam.

Bardon, Franz. *Initiation Into the Hermetics*. Wuppertal, W. Germany: Dieter Ruggeberg.

Regardie, Israel. *The Golden Dawn*. St. Paul, MN: Llewellyn.

Suzuki, Shunryu. *Zen Mind, Beginner's Mind*. New York: John Weatherhill.

Kapleau, Philip. *The Three Pillars of Zen*. New York: Doubleday.

Guenther, Herbert V. and Leslie S. Kawamura. *Mind in Buddhist Psychology*. Emeryville, CA: Dharma Publishing.

Takakusu, Junjiro. *The Essentials of Buddhist Philosophy*. York Beach, ME: Samuel Weiser. Now out of print.

Luk, Charles (Lu K'uan Yu). *The Secrets of Chinese Meditation*. York Beach, ME: Samuel Weiser; and London: Rider & Co.

Conze, Edward. *Buddhist Meditation*. New York: Harper & Row.

Ramatherio, Sri. *Unto Thee I Grant*. San Jose, CA: A.M.O.R.C.

Chang, Garma C.C. *Teachings of Tibetan Yoga*. Secaucus, NJ: Citadel Press.

Gyatso, Geshe Kelsang. Translated by Tenzin Norbu. *Clear Light of Bliss: Mahamudra in Vajrayana Buddhism*. Boston: Wisdom Publications.

Ming, Yang Jwing. *Tai Chi Chuan*. Hollywood, CA: Unique Publications.

Chia, Mantak. *Awaken Healing Energy through the Tao*. Santa Fe, NM: Aurora Press.

Hwa, Jou Tsung. *The Tao of Meditation*. Piscataway, NJ: Tai Chi Foundation.

Luk, Charles (Lu K'uan Yu). *Taoist Yoga: The Alchemy of Immortality*. York Beach, ME: Samuel Weiser; and London: Rider & Co.

Cleary, Thomas, tr. *The Taoist I Ching*. Boston: Shambhala.

Wing, R. L. tr. *The Tao of Power* (Tao Te Ching). New York: Doubleday.

Moinuddin, Hakim. *The Book of Sufi Healing*. Rochester, VT: Inner Traditions.

Khan, Hazrat Inayat. *Mastery Through Accomplishment*. New Lebanon, NY: Sufi Order Publications.

Khan, Hazrat Inayat. *Sufi Message* Volumes 1–13. New Lebanon, NY: Sufi Order Publications.

Shah, Idries. *The Sufis*. New York: Doubleday.

Timmermans, Felix. *The Perfect Joy of Saint Francis*. New York: Doubleday.

Jones, Franklin Albert. *The Spiritual Instructions of Saint Seraphim of Sarov*. Lower Lake, CA: Dawn Horse Press.

Kempis, Thomas A. *The Imitation of Christ*. New York: Doubleday.

Puhl, Louis J. *Spiritual Exercises of St. Ignatius*. Westminster, MD: Newman Press.

Chan, K. C. *More Precious Than Rubies: Handbook of Spiritual Exercises*. New York: Vantage Press.

Goldsmith, Joel. *The Infinite Way*. Marina del Rey, CA: DeVorss.

Pixley, Olive C. B. *The Armour of Light (Part I and II)*. Cheltenham, England: Helios Books. Now out of print.

Wedgwood, James Ingall. *New Insights Into Christian Worship*. Ojai, CA: St. Alban Press.

Leadbeater, C. W. *The Science of Sacraments*. Wheaton, IL: Theosophical Publishing House.

Knight, Gareth. *A Practical Guide to Qabalistic Symbolism*. York Beach, ME: Samuel Weiser.

———. *Experience of the Inner Worlds*. Cheltenham, England: Helios Books. Now out of print.

Schutz, Albert L. and Hilda W. de Schaps. *Kosher Yoga*. Quantal Publishing.

Kaplan, Aryeh. *Meditation and Kabbalah*. York Beach, ME: Samuel Weiser.

———. *Meditation and the Bible*. York Beach, ME: Samuel Weiser.

THE LORD BUDDHA HAS SAID

Let us inspect our thoughts that we do no unwholesome deed; for as we sow, so shall we reap.

Hatreds never cease by hatreds in this world. By love alone they cease. This is an ancient law.

Goodwill towards all beings is the true religion: cherish in your hearts boundless goodwill to all that lives.

Go and do your duty: show kindness to thy brothers and free them from suffering.

THE LORD CHRIST HAS SAID

So every good tree bears good fruit; but a bad tree bears bad fruit. A good tree cannot bear bad fruit, neither can a bad tree bear good fruit. . . . Thus by their fruit you will know them.

Matthew 7:17–20

"Love your enemies, do good to those who hate you, bless those who curse you, pray for those who mistreat you."

Luke 6:27–28

Love the Lord your God with all your heart and with all your soul and with all your mind. This is the first and greatest commandment. And the second is like it: Love your neighbor as yourself.

Matthew 22:37–39

Go and heal the sick.

Matthew 10:8

INDEX